OWNING MEDICAL PRACTICES

Best Practices for Sustainable Results

MARC D. HALLEY, MBA

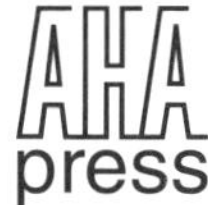

HEALTH FORUM, INC.
An American Hospital Association Company
Chicago

Printed in the United States of America

ISBN: 978-1-55648-377-6 Item Number: 164010

Project Manager: Joyce Dunne
Editorial Assistant: Barbara Novosel
Layout and Typesetting: Fine Print, Ltd.
Cover Design: Tim Kaage
Production Manager: Martin Weitzel
Acquisitions and Development: Richard Hill

Library of Congress Cataloging-in-Publication Data
Halley, Marc D.
Owning medical practices : best practices for sustainable results / Marc D. Halley.
p. ; cm.
Includes bibliographical references and index.
ISBN 978-1-55648-377-6 (alk. paper)
1. Medicine—Practice—Economic aspects. 2. Medical offices—Management.
3. Medical care—Marketing. I. Title.
[DNLM: 1. Practice Management, Medical. W 80]
R728.H32 2011
610.68—dc22 2010034616

To the team at
The Halley Consulting Group, LLC

and to our clients,
from whom we have learned these principles

Contents

List of Figures and Tables

About the Author

Marc D. Halley is president and chief executive officer of The Halley Consulting Group, LLC, Westerville, Ohio. He has provided management and consulting services to medical practices for more than twenty-five years and has worked with a variety of specialties, including hospital-owned medical practice networks across the United States. He has negotiated numerous contracts to acquire medical practices on behalf of hospitals in highly competitive environments; served as senior operating officer of primary care and multispecialty physician networks; facilitated the financial turnarounds of hospital-owned medical practice networks; and worked with physicians to take primary care networks into risk-sharing arrangements, including payer contract negotiations.

Mr. Halley developed and implemented the Best Practice Council model to engage employed physicians and hospital executives in effective operational governance. His Physician Integration Economics model has facilitated physician-hospital integration discussions across the United States. He also developed and implemented numerous tools to assist physicians and managers in tracking and improving medical practice operations. His Supervisory Training Program has been taught to medical office managers around the country.

Mr. Halley is a frequently requested speaker, having addressed governing boards, senior executives, physician groups, management teams, and national organizations, including the American College of Healthcare Executives (ACHE), the Healthcare Financial Management Association, the Medical Group Management Association, state hospital associations, The Healthcare Roundtable, The Governance Institute, and many more. He has authored and co-authored several articles that have been published in industry journals such as *Healthcare Financial Management,* the *Journal of Medical Practice Management,* and *Group Practice Journal.*

Mr. Halley's first book, *The Primary Care–Market Share Connection: How Hospitals Achieve Competitive Advantage,* was published by Health Administration Press in March 2007 as part of the ACHE Management Series imprint. He also contributed to a three-volume set titled *The Business of Healthcare,* edited by Kenneth H. Cohn and Douglas E. Hough, published in December 2007 by the Greenwood Publishing Group under the Praeger Perspectives imprint. He was also a contributor to and co-editor of *The Medical Practice Start-Up Guide,* published by Greenbranch Publishing in August 2008.

Mr. Halley has authored a self-study course titled *Building and Maintaining Referral Relationships,* which is offered by ACHE. This course is part of the ACHE advancement and recertification program.

He received his bachelor of science degree in business administration—management from Weber State University, Ogden, Utah, and his master of business administration degree from Utah State University, Logan, Utah.

Preface

As of this writing, health care reform is big news. While it remains unclear exactly what the new legislation means, two factors are very clear. First, reimbursement for medical services will continue to decline. The types of providers and specialties whose "ox is gored" may vary from time to time, but overall, reimbursement for services will fall. Second, with health care expenditures currently totaling 16 percent of gross domestic product, the industry remains very visible—uncomfortably visible—to regulators. We know that visibility leads to increased scrutiny, and increased scrutiny leads to increased regulation, which drives up the cost of doing business. We also know that demographic trends will ensure continued increase in demand for medical services over the next several decades, placing additional pressure on payers and providers alike. Consequently, health care will be front and center on the national agenda for years to come.

During the last thirty years, hospital executives have experienced a variety of changes triggered by new technology, industry consolidation, increased competition from large health systems, loss of revenues to their own medical staffs, downward pressure on reimbursement, a shift from inpatient to outpatient services dominance, new regulations, limited services providers such as ambulatory surgery centers, alternative sources of capital, and more. Still, hospitals continue to hold the key to the success of community health systems. They remain a critical workshop for the sickest patients, and they are a major source of the capital that is required by local economies to meet community need for their populations' medical care.

The last thirty years have also seen a huge shift in the disposition and objectives of physicians graduating from residencies and fellowship training programs. These highly trained young physicians have a different mental model about medicine than many of their predecessors. Rather than viewing the practice of medicine as a calling or life's mission with its never-ending demands, recent graduates often see it as a "job." Quality of life outside of work has become a significant factor in decisions made by younger physicians. Most prefer an employment option, with plenty of paid vacation time and compensation adequate to fund that vacation.

More recently, older, established physicians have begun to tire of the entrepreneurship battle. Bank loans, a major source of capital for even the largest medical practices, are no longer readily available since the onset of the 2008–2010 recession. Furthermore, the younger physicians in the group practice have no intention of becoming practice partners and buying out the older physicians so they can retire. These younger associates are in complete acceptance of long-term employment. Consequently, more established physician partners in almost all specialties are turning to hospitals to cash out their assets so they can become employed or retire (or both).

Most hospitals are likely to own medical practices and to employ physicians in a variety of specialties. This employment trend is not likely to change, even with hospitals experiencing mounting financial losses. Whether or not hospitals and physicians learn how to truly integrate, the hospital employment model is likely here to stay.

Many hospital executives are beginning to realize that they can no longer be "plant managers," viewing the hospital as the center of the universe. Having been a hospital vice president and a local health system executive vice president, I can appreciate the challenge of shifting our mind-set from that of a hospital executive to what I call a "market manager." However, in order to achieve a sustainable competitive advantage, hospital executives will need to ensure that they have adequate numbers of affiliated primary care physicians to capture the market share necessary to support the right specialty physicians operating effectively within the right hospital service lines. Whether those physicians are employed by or closely affiliated with the hospital is perhaps less important than is their willingness to work together to accomplish the following five business imperatives:[1]

1. To control market share, which is captured in primary care practices and must be attracted by affiliated specialists and hospitals
2. To demonstrate quality in terms of clinical care and service level
3. To access the capital needed for reinvestment in the entire integrated delivery system
4. To increase productivity, efficiency, and effectiveness to offset reduced reimbursement
5. To increase the rigor associated with running the business side of health care

Employing all or part of an active medical staff can potentially facilitate addressing these five business imperatives. But employing physicians and owning medical practices are not for the faint of heart.

I was taught a great lesson many years ago in a business statistics class. The professor sensed our anxiety as we tackled this complex subject. He stated: "Statistics is like a game. If you learn the rules, anyone can play well. If you don't learn the rules, you will never play well. Learn the rules." I decided to learn the rules and found that he was right; my understanding of statistics now had a solid foundation.

This book is written for those executives whose hospitals need to own medical practices and to employ physicians successfully in order to remain viable. As with understanding statistics, owning medical practices is like a game. If we learn the rules or principles for success, almost anyone can play the game. If we do not acknowledge that these practices are not hospital departments, we will have failed to learn the rules, and the enterprise will not succeed. Let's learn the rules.

Reference

1. M. Halley, "Four Business Imperatives to Manage Dynamic Change in the New Healthcare Environment," *MGMA Connexion* July (2010): 51–54.

Acknowledgments

The Halley Consulting Group, LLC, is built on six core values we strive to uphold: (1) integrity, (2) gratitude, (3) respect, (4) quality, (5) learning, and (6) tolerance. I hope this work reflects each of these values. Certainly, our search for the correct principles contained herein has helped us truly become a learning organization:

> While we possess a high level of expertise, we are a learning organization. We learn from our clients and we learn from each other. We are not afraid to ask questions or to share what we know. Ego is not an issue in our learning organization.

We have been fortunate to attract people to Halley Consulting who are (or who have become) content experts in several areas of medical practice network administration. In addition to carrying their full share of our consulting, network development, and interim management work, these experts serve one another and our clients by sharing their expertise. It is in that spirit of sharing what we know and what we have learned that this book was written.

My team and I consider the principles we identify in the following pages to be the best practices we have identified to date. Most of them are fundamentals with broad application across multiple markets with proven results. They have passed the tests of time and circumstance. These principles are modifiable according to unique market dynamics, competitive strategies, and mission objectives, but the fundamentals required to successfully own and operate a network of hospital-owned medical practices in Portland, Oregon, or Richmond, Virginia, or Baton Rouge, Louisiana, or Columbus, Ohio, are essentially the same.

This book also includes a number of our tools and models presented as figures, tables, and appendixes. These tools have been developed by our content experts to support our team and our individual clients to implement the correct principles identified herein. They have become an increasingly valuable resource over time.

Because we learn from every client and every situation, we will continue to refine our approach, our tools, and our models. Today's best practices will evolve, as well. As a team, The Halley Consulting Group is committed to documenting and sharing these principles as they evolve. Our tele-seminars, newsletter, Web page, public speaking schedule, and publications are portals for sharing what we learn from wonderful clients and skilled consultants/managers.

I express my thanks to the Halley Consulting team for contributing their experience and expertise to this work. As of this writing, that team includes Robin Walters, Jennifer Snider, Katrina Slavey, William Reiser, Lisa Reiser, Brian Morton, Pimmie Lopez, Ken Lester, Jim Hayes, Ralph Harding, Andrew Halley, Linda Forbes, Ashleigh Finley, Michael Ferry, Michele Dowdall, Kathleen Brown, Bradley Brunicardi, Karen Bridges, and Jeanette Abell, MD. Several of our team members contributed editorial comments based on their expertise. I note the specific contributions of Brian Morton to chapter 9, "Revenue Cycle Management," and of Kathleen Brown to chapter 10, "Information Technology." Lisa Reiser's ability to manage my schedule and the manuscript has been nothing short of amazing. Andrea Morgan has kept my office intact despite this and many other projects. Last, but certainly not least, I thank my wife, Debbie, and our children and grandchildren for putting up with my incessant attachment to my MacBook Pro.

Marc D. Halley, MBA
June 2010

OWNING MEDICAL PRACTICES

CHAPTER 1

The Return of Physician Employment

During the past twenty-five years, hospitals have employed significant numbers of physicians. Physician employment is one of several physician "integration" strategies and has occurred in two phases. During phase 1 (1985–1998) hospitals focused on purchasing primary care medical practices and employing primary care physicians (PCPs). Hospital executives used the employment model as a physician recruitment and start-up strategy to meet community need and to prepare for the managed care "threat." By the mid-1990s hospitals reported losing more than $80,000 per employed physician per year.[1] After 1998 most practice acquisition had ceased. Physician employment was considered a failed strategy, and some hospitals began divesting their owned medical practices. Others "pruned" their practices (code for terminating physician relationships). Still others capital starved their existing medical practice networks, creating frustration and additional physician departures—usually of the best-in-class physicians.

After a three- or four-year hiatus, physician employment by hospitals was back on the radar, and phase 2 started in late 2002; it continues as of this writing. This time around, many hospitals have employed specialists in an effort to protect or enhance revenues, particularly in their strategic service lines. As competition for referrals has increased, hospitals have responded again by hiring primary care physicians. Today, hospitals in large metropolitan areas and small rural settings offer a physician employment option and own both primary care and specialty medical practices. In fact, without an employment option, hospitals find attracting and retaining qualified physicians difficult, particularly in the primary care specialties but increasingly in invasive specialties as well.

Motives for Hospital Employment of Physicians

Both hospitals and physicians are seeking to integrate during phase 2. Physicians' motives to do so, which are facilitating the growth of hospital employment, include the following:

- *Medical malpractice premiums.* In some states (e.g., Pennsylvania, Illinois) medical malpractice premiums have become unmanageable for several private practice specialties.

- *Changes in technology*. Advances and changes in technology have affected some specialties. Consider the impact invasive cardiology has had on the incomes of heart surgeons: Drug-eluting stents placed in patients by cardiologists have reduced the number of cases that flow to surgeons.
- *Declining reimbursement*. Continued downward pressure on reimbursement for specialty services as well as primary care has increased the challenge of maintaining viable private practices.
- *Physician preference*. Physicians now leaving medical training programs indicate they prefer employment over entrepreneurship. Many carry significant debt from borrowing to finance their education and are not interested in the traditional income guarantees offered by hospitals, even when they include offers of loan forgiveness. In addition, many new physicians seek a balanced work-home life or do not adhere to the same work ethic as their predecessors. These preferences are increasingly inconsistent with viable private practice, for which productivity approaching the 75th percentile is increasingly required.
- *High-demand specialties*. Private practicing physicians and single-specialty groups are not able to match employment salary offers made by hospitals for new physicians, particularly in high-demand specialties, which contend with regional or national competition.
- *Administrative complexity*. The challenge and risk of managing the business side of medical practices continue to increase. Some physicians seek to eliminate that complexity in their current practice situation or avoid it altogether.

Motives of hospitals to employ physicians include the following:

- *Service line preservation*. Preserving, developing, or enhancing service lines is a major motivator driving the employment of specialty physicians. Some hospitals employ specialists to contend more effectively with competing hospitals' service lines or with ambulatory surgery centers. Others use specialty employment as a strategy to preserve call coverage for critical specialties. Employment is also used as a tactic to provide focused service line clinical leadership.
- *Capturing market share*. Hospitals, particularly those in competitive markets, that divested their primary care networks during phase 1 employment soon realized they were losing market share (admissions and other referrals) to competitors that controlled more primary care practices. In recent years some hospitals have required their employed primary care physicians to "refer domestic" (refer only to affiliated specialists and facilities). Even the market leaders have had a difficult time combating

such tactics and have been forced to enter the primary care business to protect or enhance their market share and market potential.

- *Attracting market share.* Some hospital executives have mistakenly felt that hiring surgeons would automatically capture market share (another form of "if we build it, they will come"). They have been disappointed to see their very expensive specialty physician resources receiving very few cases. More astute executives have recognized that hiring specialty physicians only provides capacity to attract market share from referring physicians. Further, they have realized that such referral relationships can no longer be left to chance, but must be actively and continuously nurtured.

Regardless of these and other motivations, more and more physicians prefer hospital employment, and increasing numbers of hospitals are offering those employment opportunities. Hospitals in both major metropolitan areas and rural settings have embraced employment as their principle physician recruitment and retention strategy. Physician preference and industry trends ensure that this tactic will continue to be used.

Common Mistakes in Practice Acquisition

During phase 1 of the physician employment era, hospitals consistently ignored the fact that medical practices are not hospitals or hospital departments. The rules for success in the medical practice business differ from those in hospital settings. Ignoring those rules contributed to the late 1990s declaration that physician employment was a failed strategy. Subsequent experience, however, appears to have validated the strategy as viable and implicated its poor implementation during phase 1 in its failure.

Unfortunately, some hospitals and some physicians are making the same implementation mistakes that were seen during the first phase of physician employment. These implementation errors proved costly during phase 1 and will be costly again if not addressed in phase 2.

In general, during the first phase, hospital executives misunderstood the difference between "hospital strategy" and "integration strategy." Hospital chief executive officers (CEOs) viewed themselves as hospital administrators rather than as *market managers*. They worried more about admissions and surgeries than about capturing the market share and attracting current and future referrals that would lead to those admissions and surgeries. In short, hospital CEOs failed to integrate the components of a successful integration strategy.

They did not capture market share in viable or sustainable primary care practices. They failed to consistently link their primary care physicians with accessible specialty physicians who understood that PCPs are their *most* important customers. Significantly, they failed to consistently link PCPs and specialists with accessible hospital services and responsive hospital-based physicians. Rather than capturing and attracting referrals, CEOs built capacity assuming that something or someone would fill it. They left referral relationships to chance; sometimes they won, and sometimes they lost.

They also made several tactical errors during phase 1. The most common blunders, listed below, are discussed in the paragraphs that follow.

- Hospitals paid too much for physician practices.
- Hospitals overbuilt primary care capacity.
- Hospitals removed ancillary services from the practices.
- Hospital-sponsored physician compensation models removed productivity incentives.
- Hospital employee benefits increased practice employment costs.
- New or remodeled facilities added to practice occupancy costs.
- Hospital executives disengaged the physicians from governance of the practices.
- Hospitals hired inadequate and/or inexperienced management personnel.
- Hospitals provided inadequate management systems and tools.
- Hospitals misunderstood the basics of physician integration.
- Hospitals thought they could make up practice losses on downstream hospital revenues.
- Hospitals tolerated a culture of no accountability.

Paying Too Much for Physician Practices

During phase 1, hospitals paid significant amounts of money for the goodwill value of primary care practices. This goodwill was usually amortized over a few years, an approach that wreaked havoc on medical practice income statements and contributed to the frustration of physicians and board members alike. Practice acquisition and physician employment were often "me too" strategies in competitive markets, creating bidding wars between hospital competitors (and some publicly traded physician practice management companies) and artificially driving up the fair market value of target practices based on each succeeding offer.

Overbuilding Primary Care Capacity

Hospital competitors, each seeing the same community need data, simultaneously added new primary care capacity to the same markets. In some metropolitan areas this uptick in physician capacity exceeded the demand for services, particularly for choice geographic targets, making it difficult for new practices to reach viability. With only limited understanding of how primary care practices attract patients and little analysis of local market segments (neighborhoods), hospital executives opened new practices and recruited new physicians.

Removing Ancillary Services

Hospitals routinely stripped out existing ancillary services or failed to add ancillary services usually found in small group practices. This blunder created two significant problems. First, hospitals disappointed their customers, who expected to access basic laboratory and radiology services in a convenient and accessible one-stop shop. Second, by eliminating ancillaries, hospitals removed 15–25 percent of the traditional net revenue found in successful private practices. Full practices were unable to compensate for that lost net revenue through additional cognitive services alone. The rationale for this common hospital tactic was to increase the potential for improved reimbursement at the hospital level and additional revenue to the hospital's bottom line. But at what cost? Patients were dissatisfied, and practices lost even more money, requiring additional infusions of capital from the hospital.

Decreasing Productivity Incentives and Capacity

Frequently, physicians were seeking hospital employment to secure their incomes. Many hospitals accommodated this desire by offering high base salaries with limited incentives to be productive. Many of the salary offers were more generous than the incomes physicians had experienced in private practice, and physicians gained benefits packages, including funded retirement plans. Often the incentive thresholds were set so high as to be impractical. As many physicians moved from the traditional private practice "eat what you treat" compensation approach to a high base salary model, their incentive to work declined. In addition, some physicians left private practice for employment so they could "slow down" and enjoy a more balanced lifestyle. Some younger physicians brought a different work ethic from that of preceding generations of physicians, opting for part-time employment in some cases. More women physicians were juggling work and family obligations. As a result of these and other factors, employed physician capacity and productivity fell significantly.

Increasing Practice Employment Costs

Another major motivator for physicians to sell their practices was to provide improved employee benefits to themselves and their support staff members. While some hospitals developed different (lesser) benefits packages for their owned medical practices than for the hospital itself, most treated their practices like any other department of the hospital and offered full hospital benefits to all employees. Ethical considerations, perceived fairness, ease of administration, and other reasons were an easy sell to hospital leaders, and without question the practice employees benefited from this generous offer—in the short term. Unfortunately, the medical practice business model cannot support the benefits levels routinely provided to hospital employees, and the generosity guaranteed financial losses in the practices.

Increasing Practice Occupancy Costs

Hospitals frequently agreed to provide new or remodeled office space for the medical practices they purchased or those they started from scratch. Soon, primary care practices that had been viable in space costing $10 to $15 per square foot per year were located in new or remodeled space costing $20 to $25 or more per square foot. Occupancy costs, which previously totaled 8 percent of net revenue, now consumed 15 percent. In addition, while private medical practices were forced, by their inability to accumulate capital, to add space incrementally, many hospitals pursued their traditional "build it and they will come" model, building or leasing space to accommodate planned growth. Placing two employed physicians in 10,000 square feet of space (enough for six to eight primary care physicians, depending on the office schedule) and charging the full lease cost to that cost center was not uncommon.

Disengaging the Physicians from Governance

Some hospital executives viewed physicians as employees rather than as business partners. They disengaged these valuable human resources from business decision making in the practice setting. They failed to include employed physicians in developing medical practice network strategy or in forming policies that would affect physicians' work lives. Consequently, employed physicians became "technicians" working for a paycheck rather than "owners" in the success of the enterprise.

Hiring Inadequate/Inexperienced Management Personnel

Instead of hiring an experienced medical practice network executive, many hospitals assigned a bright assistant hospital administrator to lead the practices. These young executives learned the hard way the differences between hospital and medical practice network administration. This on-the-job training process created frustration for all involved. A few hospitals sought and hired a group practice administrator to manage their networks. Some of these experienced administrators failed to make the transition from group practice administration, with its single culture and physician governance, to a network, with multiple sites and cultures operating within a hospital bureaucracy.

Providing Inadequate Management Systems and Tools

Because appreciation for the differences between the medical practice and hospital businesses was limited, many hospital-centric organizations focused their energies on financial reporting to hospital boards rather than on managerial accounting to improve performance. Medical practice income statements were developed using a hospital footprint rather than one comparable to medical practice benchmarks. Additionally, practice management system decisions were sometimes made by the hospital's software vendor, which offered a practice management system as a sideline, rather than making the best decision for the medical practice network, sacrificing service and efficiency for the entire medical practice network and its customers.

Misunderstanding the Basics of Physician Integration

Most hospital executives entered the medical practice business without understanding the basics of successful physician employment and integration. They did not invest the same effort to understand and implement critical success factors (discussed later) in this new business line as they did in the hospital business. Most hospitals had no primary care "retail" strategy guiding the placement of practices. Even fewer placed any emphasis on actively managing referral relationships between primary care physicians and affiliated specialists or hospital services.

Thinking the Hospital Could "Make Up" the Losses

In the early days of phase 1, hospital CEOs thought they would make up any losses they experienced in their hospital-owned medical practices by driving additional volume through the capital-generating engine—the hospital. While the theory seemed logical, two key factors impeded their success. First, many of the practices purchased by hospitals were at capacity and already admitted the practices' patients to the hospital directly or through referrals to the hospital's affiliated specialists. Hospital leaders were buying market share that they were already receiving—and paying too much for it—rather than investing in incremental business. Second, they failed to anticipate the capital required to cover the significant losses created by misunderstanding and mismanaging the established medical practices they purchased. Further, they failed to anticipate the level of capital needed to start new practices to capture incremental volume.

Tolerating a Culture of No Accountability

Importantly, hospital executives had a difficult time holding employed physicians accountable for performance and behavior. Traditional medical staff models had failed to create significant levels of accountability, and that lack of accountability was perpetuated by the high-base-salary compensation models that were implemented. Hospitals established very few, if any, performance expectations, and many employed physicians were totally unaware of the losses being generated by their previously viable medical practices. Worse, during the acquisition process, many hospital leaders set the expectations for the selling physicians that "nothing would change" in the practices purchased.

While some hospital executives learned valuable lessons from their phase 1 experience, many are making the same or similar mistakes in phase 2. New executives are attempting physician integration for the first time. To CEOs' credit, as of this writing, most hospitals are no longer paying for goodwill for practices they acquire; most are purchasing fixed assets only. A few hospital executives are actively engaging employed physicians in leadership roles for hospital-owned medical practice networks. Several hospitals are pursuing experienced executives to manage their networks. Still, as a general rule, hospital executives are making some of the same significant and avoidable blunders as they employ primary care and specialty physicians in phase 2.

Practice Acquisition—Not for the Faint of Heart

Owning medical practices and employing physicians is not an endeavor to be undertaken lightly. Investment in a "cold start"[2] family practice (one in which a new physician is established in a new location), for example, can routinely reach $500,000 per physician in recruitment costs and operating losses while the practice matures. New specialty practices can reach financial viability relatively quickly if adequate primary care referrals are attracted, but operating losses driven by large specialty salaries can occur for a year or more. Acquisition of existing practices can also consume significant amounts of capital. If they are structured properly, however, established practices should not experience much operating loss during a transition to hospital ownership. Under any circumstances, a physician integration strategy that includes practice ownership is a significant financial commitment.

In addition to the financial commitment required to acquire or start medical practices, the ongoing energy and focus required to successfully *maintain* a network of hospital-owned medical practices is significant. This commitment of energy starts in the C-suite and requires the time and attention of the hospital CEO and other senior executives, who need to understand the rules for success in the medical practice business as well as they understand the critical success factors for the hospital enterprise. Without this energy and senior-level commitment, the owned network will never achieve its potential.

The CEO must view himself or herself as a market manager rather than as a hospital administrator, as discussed earlier. The chief financial officer (CFO), in addition to allocating adequate capital to the network, must ensure that network leadership—executives and physicians—has proper managerial accounting information, including a realistic budget, to adequately benchmark and measure performance. The senior human resources officer must acknowledge the differences inherent in the medical practice business and develop relevant policies and procedures to help guarantee the success of this unique business, rather than simply imposing "hospital policy" on the physician network. The chief information officer cannot hide behind the hospital's commitment to a single software vendor. Instead, he or she needs to work with network management to select practice management and electronic medical record software that will support, as a priority, those staff and practitioners "in the field" as well as the enterprise's objectives.

Successful ownership of medical practices starts with a clear understanding of *physician integration economics* (PIE). Physician integration economics defines how market share is captured and held in primary care practices, which are "the doctor" for most households. It illustrates how the primary care market share generates revenue in PCP practices up to the point at which patients require specialty or hospital services. The PIE model further shows how PCPs and their staff members make the majority of referrals to specialty physicians, where additional revenue is generated for services rendered. Importantly, the model demonstrates how patient referrals (market share referrals) are sent from PCPs directly or through specialty physicians to hospitals, where specialists help generate relatively large amounts of hospital revenue, some of which becomes capital for future investment. Figure 1-1 illustrates how the wise CEO (again, referred to as a market manager rather than as a hospital administrator) preserves and reinvests capital to strengthen all components of the integrated system. Ensuring that affiliated primary care practices capture and retain adequate market share and that affiliated specialists and hospitals can and do attract that market share becomes the major focus of every successful CEO–market manager.

Those hospital strategists who choose to use medical practice ownership and physician employment as an integration strategy, and who do so successfully, can achieve a sustainable competitive advantage. However, meeting the challenge of successfully investing in and maintaining a physician employment strategy requires the very best effort by both physician leaders and hospital leaders. The strategy must be based on a clear understanding of what Peter Drucker calls "the theory of the business,"[3] which includes a firm grasp of *correct principles*—the theory of the medical practice business (described later and referred to throughout the book)—driving success in any enterprise. Senior hospital leaders must be willing to invest in and participate with the experienced leadership (including physicians) necessary to ensure successful implementation of correct principles on both network-wide and practice-specific bases.

Figure 1-1. Physician Integration Economics

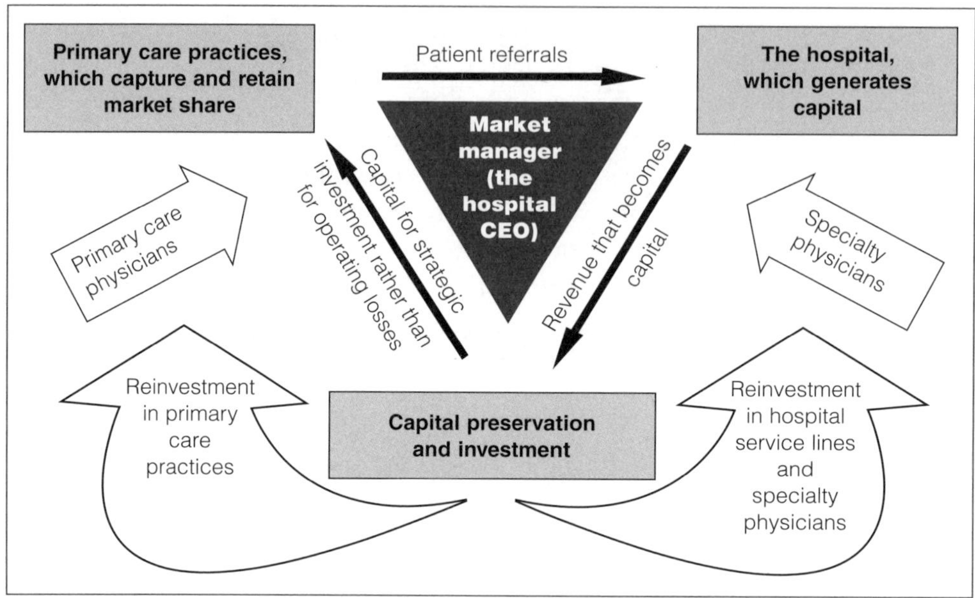

Source: The Halley Consulting Group, LLC (www.halleyconsulting.com), copyright © 2008. Adapted with permission.

The team at The Halley Consulting Group has spent years creating operating plans for new hospital-owned medical practice networks and evaluating established hospital-owned physician networks to improve performance. In the process we have developed a set of best practices based on correct operating principles that have worked in multiple markets and settings in several parts of the United States.

A few of our clients have initially struggled with the notion of *best practice,* fearing that we would provide a "canned" solution for their unique markets. Each market is distinct, as are the strategic responses of our client hospitals. However, certain tried-and-true operating principles consistently produce a successful outcome in a family medicine practice, whether located in Portland, Oregon, or Lumberton, North Carolina, and certain medical practice *network* operating principles consistently work in locations ranging from Baton Rouge, Louisiana, to Clinton, Iowa. These operating principles are categorized in twelve areas of business administration, ranging from effective operational governance and decision making to practice operations management to performance measurement. Those principles that have stood the test of both time and circumstance become best practices and are the subject of this text.

A summary of the principles in each area of business administration follows, and subsequent chapters explore these concepts and their implementation. Will these principles evolve over time? Of course they will, as circumstances change in medical practices. These are, however, the best practices we have identified to date.

Critical Success Factors

We refer to the following principles as *critical success factors* in physician employment. We do so because, in our experience, failure to address each area properly is highly correlated with poor performance. Effective implementation, on the other hand, is highly correlated with success.

The sections below discuss critical success factors in each of the following categories:

- An understanding of the theory of the medical practice business
- The building of a hospital-owned medical practice network
- Operational governance
- Management infrastructure
- Practice and network promotion
- Human resource management
- Network and practice operations
- Revenue cycle management
- Information technology
- Physical facilities and equipment
- Finance and accounting
- A culture of accountability

Understanding the Theory of the Business

Although McDonald's, the hamburger chain, and Ruth's Chris Steak House are both restaurant businesses, it is unlikely that a Ruth's Chris waiter would invite us to have fries and a drink with our burger. The rules for success in each setting differ. Failure to observe those rules guarantees failure to succeed in that setting.

While it seems intuitive, hospital executives do not always apply this logic to their ownership of medical practices. A medical practice and a hospital are both in the health care business, but the rules for success in one do not necessarily apply to the other. A classic example is the common practice of imposing a hiring freeze "across the board." The hiring freeze is a commonly used tactic in the hospital business, where fixed costs make up about 50 percent of the cost structure. Cutting labor and other variable costs can, indeed, drive a hospital back to achieving budget. The same does not apply to a medical practice, for which the majority of costs are human resources—70–80 percent, depending on the specialty—which are "fixed" costs in the short term. The next highest cost is building occupancy, which is usually less than 10 percent of the cost structure, again depending on the specialty.

While controlling labor costs is certainly important, the only way to achieve success in a medical practice is by driving volume and revenue. The chief source of that volume and revenue is a *productive* physician who does what only a physician can do and delegates everything else to less expensive support staff. Hiring freezes or hiring delays in a medical practice reduce the productivity of its most expensive resource (the physician) and exacerbate rather than correct performance issues. Understanding these differences and other important rules for success is critical for hospital executives as they work with physician leaders to implement a hospital-owned medical practice strategy.

It is also important for physician and administrative leaders to understand that owning and managing several practice locations distributed geographically—a *network*—is not the same as managing a group practice with departments located in different hallways of a facility. Every location is a unique culture, whether we acknowledge it or not. Even hospital-owned practices started from scratch differ from one another because each is characterized by its individual physicians, support staff, and manager. Developing standards in such a setting must be limited to critical issues (e.g., a common electronic medical record, the employee benefits package), with more autonomy given to practices as they address their unique markets, physician practice styles and personalities, customer base, physical facility, and so forth.

Building a Hospital-Owned Medical Practice Network

In addition to operating principles, hospital and physician leaders must understand physician integration economics, which should drive the development and growth of a hospital-owned medical practice network. Network development planning starts with the end user, or what we call the "retail customer," and includes *retail analysis*.[4] A complete understanding of how women make health care decisions for their personal care and that of their families, including where, how, and why they select primary care physicians, should guide our planning.

For example, primary care physician selections for the family tend to center around homes and schools, and access is a key issue for patients, especially with more than half of U.S. women currently in the work force. Understanding these and related factors should drive the development of the primary care component of the hospital's network, including primary care specialties such as family medicine, internal medicine (IM), pediatrics, IM/pediatrics, and obstetrics; locations; ancillary services available; and hours of operation. These primary care physicians and locations capture, serve, and retain market share up to the point at which the patient requires additional services.

Once the hospital's target primary care locations and services are identified, the organization should determine which specialists will be necessary to support the primary care network, some or all of whom may be employed by the hospital, as well. This decision is usually dictated by current or anticipated demand from the affiliated primary care physicians (employed or otherwise) and their patients, both of whom are critical customers, as well as the service line objectives of the organization's affiliated hospitals. Although more and more hospitals have contract terms requiring primary care physicians to refer domestic, it is far better to *attract* than to *mandate* patient referrals by becoming the specialist of choice[5] and the hospital of choice.

Operational Governance

Perhaps *the* major blunder hospital executives make upon entering the business of owning medical practices is failing to engage the employed physicians as partners in the success of the network and their individual practices. The council approach to governance corrects this problem. Operational governance includes establishing a compelling vision in support of the larger entity, identifying strategies to support that vision, establishing relevant policies and procedures to guide daily operations, monitoring performance, holding employed physicians accountable to perform, and holding the implementation team (management team) accountable to ensure the success of *every willing physician*.

Operational governance occurs at two levels: the network and the practice site. A network operations council (NOC) is responsible for network-wide initiatives in support of the integrated delivery system. The NOC usually includes up to six employed physicians (one of whom is the chairperson) and three hospital executives (including the hospital executive who signs the physician employment contracts) and is responsible for the ultimate success of the network as a whole.

Each practice in the network has a practice operations council (POC), which is responsible for site-specific initiatives and the ultimate success of the practice. In most network practices, every physician and other provider is a member of the POC.

An appropriate operational governance model engages physicians in setting strategic direction and establishing policies that affect their ability to provide quality care in a caring environment. Properly functioning operations councils have also proven effective in holding physicians accountable for their performance.

Operational governance councils subject all of their decisions to the following four *critical success filters*:

1. Does the policy or decision under consideration maintain or enhance clinical quality, as defined by our physicians?
2. Does the policy or decision under consideration maintain or enhance service quality, as defined by our patients and their referring physicians?
3. Does the policy or decision under consideration maintain or enhance physician (or other provider) productivity?
4. Does the policy or decision under consideration maintain or enhance practice operational and financial viability?

Any issue that cannot adequately address all four filters is tabled for modification or turned down.

Management Infrastructure

An implementation team works under the direction of the NOC and the POCs to implement strategy and policy as developed by both operations councils. The management team holds staff members accountable to support every willing physician to provide high-quality clinical care in a caring manner. Managers do not hold physicians accountable; this accountability is enforced by the operations councils.

Medical directors or physician/administrator dyads, which have not proven to be effective management models, are not necessary. Instead, network executives and managers are selected for their ability to provide implementation leadership and manage daily operations successfully.

The management team structure usually matches the operational governance model: A network executive is accountable to the NOC; a practice manager is accountable to each POC. Some additional infrastructure is also required at the network level, but the management team's focus is on building bench strength and teamwork in the practices.

Practice and Network Promotion

Promotion should be driven by the leadership's knowledge of the customer. Because women still make most health care decisions for the family, they are the logical primary care practice target.[6] Furthermore, because most specialty referrals are made or influenced by primary care physicians, they are the logical target for specialists and hospitals seeking those referrals for their employed specialists.

The majority of new patients select a primary care physician based on a referral from a friend or relative who is an established patient. Consequently, while newspaper advertising and direct mail marketing campaigns are great ways to start promoting a new primary care practice, excellent customer service is the best approach to promoting a primary care practice in the long term.[7] That high level of service yields happy patients, who literally become a passive sales force on behalf of the practice.[8]

While specialists must treat referred patients with high-quality clinical care and caring, specialty practice promotion also involves addressing the needs, wants, and priorities of referring physicians and other providers. In short, patient "referrals follow relationships," and "all relationships atrophy over time."[9]

Human Resource Management

Physicians and support staff usually account for 70 percent or more of the cost structure of a medical practice. For this reason, decisions affecting compensation and benefits costs for these human resources are critical elements of a winning hospital-owned network strategy.

Successful physician compensation models, like successful "eat what you treat" private practice models, must promote and reward patient volume and practice revenue. Clinical and service quality factors can also be considered, although paying a licensed professional extra to provide high-quality, as opposed to average or low-quality, clinical care smacks of ignorance on the part of management. If a provider does not want to comply with the practice's performance standards, she should be replaced rather than rewarded.

Support staff wage ranges must be competitive with the local medical practice business and, for business staff, with organizations offering similar positions (e.g., receptionists, cashiers, billers, office managers). Most hospital benefits packages are not sustainable in a medical practice setting. Indeed, hospitals themselves have struggled for years with the issue of benefit equity among different business lines.

Additionally, although hospital executives sometimes choose to employ the medical practice support staff under the hospital's payroll, some human resource policies do not apply to these employees. Being smart about human resource issues in the first place by developing an effective physician compensation model, designing a sustainable employee benefits package, and identifying relevant human resource policies is the safest route to success. Needing to change models and policies after the fact is much more difficult, but it is often essential to achieve success in practice ownership.

Network and Practice Operations

Clinical quality, the service experience, physician productivity, and financial viability are all tested in the crucible of daily operations. As a first priority, customer needs, wants, and priorities and, as a second priority, physician productivity must drive the following:

- Performance expectations for every member of the team
- The way the work is organized
- The staff hired
- How staff are trained
- How staff are managed
- How performance is measured
- Individual accountability

New physicians usually see far fewer patients than do established physicians. Consequently, new physicians and their support staff have time to better understand and respond to customer (patient and referring physician) needs, wants, and priorities. As the practice becomes busier, the challenge of maintaining the service experience becomes daunting. With increased patient volume, any poorly designed practice operations process will cause frustration among customers and may even lead to the practice's demise if a more astute competitor is available. As a physician becomes busier, well-designed processes and adequate numbers of well-trained staff become essential to maintain the service levels and productivity required by his or her customers. Experience has shown that the most productive medical practices in the United States have more staff per physician than do their less productive counterparts.[10]

Revenue Cycle Management

Traditionally, many hospital executives anticipated that medical practice billing could be managed successfully in the hospital central billing office. To their chagrin, they discovered that days in accounts receivable usually increased and the collection percentage fell as a result. Why? Hospital billing, with its large balances and eventual account closure, is vastly different from medical practice billing, which is characterized by small balances and patient accounts that operate like revolving credit.

Successful revenue cycle management starts and ends in the practice site. Such critical components as gathering and verifying billing information, collecting co-payments, performing coding and documentation duties, collecting past-due balances, and making de facto credit extension to patients all fall under the purview of the practice manager rather than the billing manager.

Thriving hospital-owned networks hold the practice manager accountable for much of the revenue cycle management process. A billing office manager is held accountable to efficiently process and vigorously pursue clean primary and secondary insurance claims—even the $50 claims that a hospital billing department might routinely write off. The billing office and the practice will likely share the work of responding to patient inquiries, based on who gets the patient call first.

Information Technology

Like all decisions at the medical practice network or practice site, information technology decisions should meet all four critical success filters, enumerated earlier. Practice management system and electronic medical records software decisions should be based *first* on the needs of the practice and second on compatibility with hospital systems and ease of support.

Care should be taken not to automatically install the practice management software the hospital's existing vendor has designed as a sideline. Some of these packages have proven unfriendly for users and, in turn, frustrating for customers.

Some of the most successful integrated systems employ innovative technology experts who focus first on helping their owned medical practices efficiently meet the needs, wants, and priorities of their customers. They place secondary focus on integrating that technology throughout the system, as needed. Best practice organizations have both technical experts and training experts dedicated to the technology employed in their hospital-owned medical practices.

Physical Facilities and Equipment

The third highest expense in a medical practice cost structure is building occupancy (behind the cost of physicians and the cost of support staff). Hospital executives routinely double building occupancy costs for their owned medical practices in pursuit of the traditional "build it and they with come" model.

Instead of investing in facilities, which sit empty while medical practice losses mount, wise executives invest in *market share* by placing primary care physicians in the right geographic locations, leasing nice, but not elaborate, facilities. Once market share has been captured, decisions can be made about "big box" and "small box" office space with expanded ancillaries and specialty physician rotation to meet the needs, wants, and priorities of referring physicians and their now established market share.

The question of ancillary services always arises with hospital-owned medical practices. Hospitals frequently remove most ancillaries from their owned practices to improve the hospital's financial picture or in pursuit of improved reimbursement on some services. This short-term thinking ignores two important facts. First, patients do not want to go to the hospital for routine laboratory, radiology, or other services. They prefer to visit a convenient, one-stop shop for all services. And because capturing and retaining market share should be the hospital CEO's top long-term priority, he or she should listen to what the patients want and act accordingly.

Second, removing ancillary services from primary care practices (or never installing them) eliminates from 15 percent to 25 percent, perhaps more, of the net patient revenue normally achieved in private practice settings. This lost revenue reduces the financial performance of hospital-owned practices, which then require additional hospital capital to cover the operating losses. Adept hospital executives provide the capital up front in the form of investment in basic ancillary services, which are appreciated by customers and create additional practice revenues to reduce operating losses.

Finance and Accounting

While financial reporting is critical to meet fiduciary responsibilities, managerial accounting is the priority for successful medical practice management. Performance reporting and indicators must be based on medical practice metrics rather than on a hospital measurement format. A dedicated accounting professional who understands the medical practice business must be engaged to ensure that

POCs and their managers have the information they need to successfully manage according to performance targets, internal comparative measures, and external benchmarks.

Chief financial officers must ensure that physicians help develop realistic budgets and then *own* them. The common practice of arbitrarily ratcheting up revenues and squeezing expenses after a realistic budget is submitted disconnects physicians from the process and invalidates the budget in their mind. Wise budget managers engage their medical professionals up front in developing stretch goals rather than imposing goals that the manager created for them, and they do so with the support of wise CFOs.

A Culture of Accountability

While physicians, staff, and managers commonly *feel responsible* for high-quality performance in a medical practice setting, it is relatively uncommon for them to actually be *held accountable* for their performance.

Creating a culture of accountability is challenging in almost every organization;[11] in those composed of professionals it may be intimidating. Variability in clinical and service quality across the health care industry and even within a medical staff provides ample evidence of poor accountability for technical and behavioral performance.

As a best practice, successful hospital-owned networks establish governance structures and clear policies regarding performance. Importantly, physician and executive leaders *act* on performance issues with the support of thoughtful physician and executive council members. Managers are held accountable on a weekly basis to perform according to specific action plans. They, in turn, hold support staff members accountable for specific performance targets. Those who cannot or do not consistently meet performance standards do not remain with the organization, regardless of the letters behind their name.

Summary

The material in the chapters that follow is based on more than twenty years of experience in starting up or improving the performance of hospital-owned medical practices and medical practice networks. The chapter topics derive from The Halley Consulting Group's formal medical practice network evaluations, which have yielded the best practices we subsequently have used in multiple network operating plans. Our experience with hands-on implementation in numerous settings over the past two decades has allowed us to see and gather the best practices presented herein.

Ownership of medical practices does not have to be a money-losing, all-consuming proposition. Hospital-employed physicians are just as capable as their private practicing peers of building and maintaining operationally and financially viable medical practices. The key, as in private practice, is to implement correct operating principles, a process that features leaders who expect high performance and engage employed physicians who are interested in partnering under those terms. Successful medical practice ownership must be based on a clear understanding that medical practices are not hospital departments. They must be managed according to the critical success factors for medical practices. Let's learn those factors.

References

1. Health Care Advisory Board, "Stopping the Bleed: Reversing Losses in Owned Practices" (Washington, DC: The Advisory Board, 1999).
2. M. Halley, *The Primary Care–Market Share Connection: How Hospitals Achieve Competitive Advantage,* 36–37 (Chicago: Health Administration Press, 2007).
3. Peter F. Drucker, "The Theory of the Business," *Harvard Business Review* 72, no. 5 (1994): 95–104.
4. Halley, *The Primary Care–Market Share Connection,* 100–105.
5. K. Cohn and D. Hough, eds., *Practice Management,* 48–51, vol. 1, *The Business of Healthcare* (Westport, CT: Praeger, 2008).
6. P. Braus, *Marketing Health Care to Women: Meeting New Demands for Products and Services,* 1 (Ithaca, NY: American Demographics, 1997).
7. Cohn and Hough, *Practice Management,* 103.
8. Halley, *The Primary Care–Market Share Connection,* 38.
9. Ibid., 120–121.
10. Matthew Vuletich, "Smooth Operators: Recipe for Better Performers Calls for Higher Productivity, Right Staffing Mix and Diligent Collections," *MGMA e-Connexion* 113 (2006) (membership login required for access).
11. M. Halley, "A Culture of Accountability: What Distinguishes an Exceptional Medical Group," *Group Practice Journal* 54, no. 3 (2005): 11–14.

CHAPTER 2

Planning Your Hospital-Owned "Network"

It has been said that physicians make poor employees. While that may be true, they also make potentially *great* business partners, even if they are on the hospital's payroll.

Employed Physicians as Partners

Physicians are what Peter Drucker calls "knowledge workers."[1] Drucker states that, unlike traditional employees who can be told what to do, how, and how fast to complete their tasks, "knowledge workers cannot be supervised effectively."[2] The descriptors associated with Drucker's knowledge workers as they apply to physicians include the following:

- Workshop
- Means of production
- Tools of production
- Continuing medical education
- Accountability
- Loyalty

Workshop

Physicians still require a "workshop" in which to provide their services. The nature of that workshop has changed with advancing technology and shifts in competitive factors. Procedures that once required an inpatient stay and a hospital operating room to be performed can now be provided in an outpatient or ambulatory setting, often one owned by the physician performing them. Many ancillary services and procedures can now be provided in the medical office as a result of improvements in technology.

Means of Production

Regardless of the workshop location, the physician still owns the means of production—his or her medical knowledge and practiced skills. The ownership of these means makes the physician, employed by the hospital or otherwise, "independent and highly mobile."[3]

Tools of Production

Assuming physicians have that knowledge and those skills, they need tools of production to act on them, particularly those physicians practicing in invasive specialties but also, increasingly, primary care physicians, especially family medicine physicians. They are requiring more sophisticated tools of production for screening and other procedures, as improved technology has made these tools available for the medical office. Often, in fact, invasive specialists may be seen assisting primary care physicians to establish screening services so that the specialists can spend more time doing the procedures that result from more accessible screening. This cycle presents a win for all parties, including patients.

Continuing Medical Education

Ongoing training is critical to maintaining and enhancing the knowledge and skills of knowledge workers. Continuing medical education requirements are usually a motivator to participate in further training, and it is an area in which a hospital should invest liberally for the benefit of the patients served, the physician, and the organization.

Accountability

A leader who supervises an employee who knows more about the subject than the leader faces a significant challenge. This scenario may be clearly seen in the working relationship between a hospital executive and a physician. But physicians, like all knowledge workers and other members of the health care team, must be held accountable for their performance.

To hold their physicians accountable, some hospital leaders have mistakenly assumed that physicians, like other employees, should answer to line managers, starting with the office manager. Experience has proven that this method does not work. Others have suggested that physicians will respond to being held accountable by other physicians. This method has clearly proven ineffective at the practice level. (No one wants to make his or her on-call partner angry, for example.)

Accountability is sometimes more effectively enforced at the network level, with the right physician leader or leadership involved. The method that has proven most effective combines the credibility of clinical leadership at the network operational governance level with the executive (physician or otherwise) who signs the physician employment contract. More on this topic is offered in chapter 3.

Loyalty

Drucker's insightful comments also help us understand why some employed physicians continue to send their referrals outside the employing organization. He states:

> [L]oyalty can no longer be obtained by the paycheck. The organization must earn loyalty by proving to its knowledge employees that it offers them exceptional opportunities for putting their knowledge to work. . . . This change reminds us that it is the individual, and especially the skilled and knowledgeable employee, who decides in large measure what he or she will contribute to the organization and how great the yield from his or her knowledge will be.[4]

Engaging physicians in the success of the organization at the practice, network, or integrated delivery level cannot be accomplished by monetary incentives or by fiat. Such engagement requires the personal attention of the hospital or integrated delivery system chief executive officer (CEO)—that is, the market manager, as described in chapter 1.

Loyalty is relationship driven. It must be nurtured over time, and it can be destroyed by one decision *perceived* to be unfair or unethical. Wise market managers (CEOs) understand that they are not the "boss" in the traditional sense. They are not generals with a team of conscripted soldiers. They are maestros who lead an orchestra of professionals in a variety of specialties, each of whom strives for perfection in his or her own realm. At the same time these professionals cannot achieve their potential as solitary entities. Organizing these knowledge workers around a coordinated musical score is essential for the success of the whole. In health care, the ultimate musical score is an integrated system of delivery wherein each member plays together and in tune with the others.

Why Create a Network?

Hospital CEOs and hospital-employed physician leaders are often heard to lament over the challenges of building a "group" mentality among the employed physicians. In larger networks, some physicians never see each other and do not know one another. The motivation to create a traditional group practice is unclear. In a multispecialty network, that incentive is largely related to the flow of referrals from primary care physicians to specialists and back again. In primary care networks it appears to derive from the desire to facilitate the standardization and management of disparate pods around the community.

Some leaders have implemented quarterly town hall meetings, which do facilitate physicians' acquaintance with one another and allow them to share innovations and clinical expertise. Others have tried internal newsletters, holiday parties, and other tactics to create that group feel. Unfortunately, most of these efforts, while beneficial in some ways, do not promote a group practice mentality.

Why? A network of individual practices, with locations on campus and around the hospital's primary and secondary service areas, is not, by definition, a group practice. It cannot be governed or managed like a group practice because it is a different species.

Several factors differentiate a *group practice* from a *network of practices,* and understanding them is an important component of the "theory of the business" for hospital-owned medical practice networks. These factors are presented in table 2-1.

These differences often thwart attempts to create a group practice mentality. However, acknowledging the differences and establishing the network using correct principles, or tenets, help fulfill the underlying objective (e.g., referral management).

Table 2-1. Factors Differentiating a Group Practice from a Network

Factor	Typical Group Practice	Typical Network
Location	A single location with all providers under the same roof	Multiple, smaller locations distributed around the hospital's service area
Culture	A single culture under the same roof	Multiple cultures driven by different locations and the physicians, manager, and staff assigned to those locations
Operational Governance	A single governing body that makes decisions for the whole	Best practice is governance at two levels (e.g., network and practice site)
Specialty Composition	May be single specialty or multispecialty under the same roof	Single-specialty pods in various locations
Financial Accountability	Sharing and subsidizing across the group practice	Practice site (cost center) accountability for performance
Management	A single manager or an executive (depending on practice size) with bottom-line accountability; executive may have department heads with budget accountability	Network executive and practice site managers each with bottom-line accountability
Referral Patterns	Hallway referrals with group financial incentive to keep patient referrals in-house in order to make payroll	Specialists work in a different cost center and must earn the referrals by becoming the "specialist of choice" (although "refer domestic" mandates are becoming more common)

The Operating Plan

We are frequently called on to assist hospitals new to the physician employment business, or those returning after a previous bad experience, in launching or rebuilding their hospital-owned networks properly. We always recommend starting with the development of an operating plan. The document itself will be a valuable reminder when times are tough of why the organization went into the business. It will also prompt the hospital leadership to stick to correct principles when they are tempted to stray from them in the name of expediency.

The most important part of an operating plan is the planning process itself. No better forum exists to engage hospital executives and physician leaders in understanding and planning to implement the theory of the business.

The following players should be included in the planning process:

- The hospital CEO
- The hospital chief financial officer (CFO)
- The hospital human resources officer
- The hospital chief information officer (CIO)
- A representative from the hospital strategic planning and business development department
- The hospital marketing and communications executive
- A representative from the hospital medical staff office
- A representative from the billing office
- Hospital and practice physician leadership

The following discussion provides detail on the roles of each player in the planning process.

The CEO

The hospital CEO is what Daryl Conner calls the "initiating sponsor."[5] He or she is the "buck stop"—the board-appointed fiduciary who has the greatest impact on strategy and capital allocation. The CEO's attendance in the planning process will confirm his or her commitment to be a market manager rather than a hospital administrator.[6] By participating, the CEO will gain intimate knowledge of practice ownership as a valuable physician integration tool and will be better prepared to engage hospital-employed physicians in the operational governance of the practice network. Importantly, the CEO's attendance and interest will facilitate the attendance and interest of everyone else on the planning team—especially those who think they are in the hospital business rather than in the business of delivering integrated health care.

The CFO

Engaging the CFO in the planning process is also critical for the success of the network. Chief financial officers usually have a great deal of influence over key issues such as managerial accounting for the practices (including appropriate general ledger categories), revenue cycle management, budgeting, and capital allocation. The CFO's interest in and influence over distributing ancillary services in the medical practices, instead of at the hospital, require his or her clear understanding of physician integration economics and where the customers want and expect those services to be offered.

The Human Resources Officer

Owning medical practices has huge implications for the human resources office. Benefits questions usually arise first in the planning process. The often automatic "give them hospital benefits" significantly affects hospital-owned practices by driving up employment costs. Human resource policies can also be an issue. For example, hospital-centric policies often call for open positions to be posted internally for a week or two before being advertised externally. This process is fine for a facility with 1,500 employees, where work can be shared across many hands in the short term. But in that solo practice with three employees, losing one staff member has the same effect as losing 500 all at once in the hospital. In addition, the human resources executive should understand the nuances of physician compensation models and be able to support and explain the principles of successful models.

The CIO

Increasingly, the hospital technology experts have significant influence on customer service and productivity in the medical office. Selecting a practice management system from a vendor with which the hospital already has a relationship is not always the best decision. Selecting an electronic medical record that addresses practice issues as well as hospital issues is essential. Consequently, the CIO is a critical member of the operational planning team.

Strategic Planning and Business Development

The senior planning and senior development officers need to participate in the operational planning process. Both of these roles and the executives who fill them are critical to the CEO's success at developing an integrated approach to the market. Coordinating all of the pieces of an integrated system often falls to these executives. Their understanding of physician integration economics and the role of the hospital-owned network is a critical component of successful implementation.

The Hospital Marketing and Communications Executive

A properly functioning hospital-owned medical practice network requires effective promotion to internal stakeholders as well as external customers. Marketing experts play a key role in developing appropriate promotion efforts for primary care practices, which differ from promotion of internal medicine subspecialties, which differs from that of more invasive specialty practices. Linking primary care with specialty physicians, and both of them with hospital services, is often another significant role for the marketing department.

The Medical Staff Office

The medical staff office and the billing office (discussed next) also need to be represented on the operations planning team. Medical staff credentialing and payer credentialing are sometimes an afterthought in developing a network of new or newly employed physicians and other providers. The process can be lengthy, resulting in frustrated physicians and financial losses. Both of these credentialing processes often use the same information, which should be shared and coordinated for maximum efficiency. Defining the process on the front end in the operating plan requires participation by a medical staff office representative.

The Billing Office

In addition to the billing office's role in payer credentialing, the central billing office manager should be engaged in the planning to help design the practice revenue cycle management process. Correct principles dictate that billing for practices should be separated from hospital billing because of the differences in the businesses. Nevertheless, having a billing expert assisting in planning for a *central processing office* is most helpful.

Physician Leadership

A hospital chief medical officer or vice president of medical affairs can provide insight based on his or her experience and specialty, but this input is usually not enough to ensure adequate planning. Participation by physicians in the development of the operating plan provides critical input into the process. Such participation, however, may present some challenges that require careful planning.

Involvement of selected private practicing physicians may create political problems or lead to the premature release of information. If a few physicians are already employed, that pool may provide valuable input if the right physicians are selected to participate. Despite the potential political risks, we usually recommend that the organization invite a few key physicians to participate in the planning process. These physicians should be leaders who can sidestep their personal agendas and help build an operating model based on correct principles. We recommend that the physicians be compensated for their participation in the planning process, which should be scheduled in a way that minimizes the impact on their daily practice schedule. It is also important to remember that most physicians have only been exposed to the group practice model. Developing a network of group practices requires a different mind-set, so the ability to conceptualize will be an important factor in the selection of physicians for the planning process.

Plan Facilitation

Once the participants have been identified, we recommend selecting one or more facilitators who can lead the planning group through discussion of several critical factors. The order of those topics is important, as they should build on one another, and a facilitator can help maintain a structured approach. The correct principles, introduced below and described in detail in the following chapters, will help guide the discussion, but their application in each market must be driven by those who are familiar with local circumstance. Note that this does not say *change the principles* but rather *guide their application.* Our boldness in this matter derives from years of experience consulting with and managing hospital-owned medical practice networks in many parts of the United States. Those practices that stick to correct principles win. Those that do not, lose—every time.

Operating plan topic priorities and the chapters in which they are discussed are as follows:

- Engaging physicians in operational governance (chapter 3)
- Management infrastructure (chapter 4)
- Network development (chapter 5)
- Practice and network marketing (chapter 6)
- Human resource management (chapter 7)
- Practice and network operations (chapter 8)
- Revenue cycle management (chapter 9)
- Information technology (chapter 10)
- Physical facilities and equipment (chapter 11)
- Finance and accounting (chapter 12)

In our experience, these topics can be adequately addressed during five or six three-hour planning sessions, with the facilitator(s) documenting portions of the plan between sessions.

Once the sessions are complete, the facilitators should develop a quarterly action plan (QAP) to drive implementation of the operating plan. The QAP documents the strategies and tactics that flow from the planning process. It identifies when those initiatives should be initiated and, where relevant, completed. The QAP also documents an assigned leader for each initiative.

The QAP is the most important accountability tool to be used by the network operations council (NOC). It allows the NOC to manage the pace of implementation and change. In addition, it reduces the tendency for private agendas to derail the implementation process.

The QAP helps maintain management's focus on the factors that are important to the success of the network. Without its guiding structure, those factors might be lost among the many urgencies of daily operations.

Basic Tenets of Planning

Before launching into the development of an operating plan, the planning group should consider several basic tenets that have proven true, even in the most complex markets, over the last twenty years. These ten tenets should undergird the entire planning process.

Tenet 1: Employed physicians, at least those you would want on your team, are just as capable as their private practice peers of achieving private practice levels of performance. In fact, private practice performance should be the gold standard against which effectiveness is measured. Most private practices break even each year while paying the physician the local market rate of compensation. Assuming they achieve the same revenues (including ancillary services) found in private practice, and assuming they incur only the expenses found in those settings, hospital-owned practices should also break even while paying the physician the local market rate. This equation is the definition of "net one" financial performance, discussed in chapter 12.

Tenet 2: The medical practice "game" is won or lost on the revenue side of the income statement. Hospitals cannot cost-cut their way to success in the medical practice business because 75 percent or more of the cost structure is human resources—cost that is fixed in the short term. Hiring freezes/delays and other Draconian cost-cutting measures routinely employed in hospitals often exacerbate performance problems in a medical practice setting. Every decision, every policy, every procedure, even in the planning process, must be made with the following eight revenue factors in mind:[7]

- Volume/capacity: Are there enough potential patients in the geographic area to match our physician and mid-level provider capacity?
- Payer mix: Do we have a sustainable payer mix in the practice?
- Fees for services: Are our fees at least as high as our highest reimbursing payer?

- Customer service: Do our practices meet the needs, wants, and priorities of our patients and their referring physicians?
- Provider productivity: Is the productivity of our physicians and mid-level providers optimized through an appropriate compensation model, effective scheduling, and adequate support staffing?
- Coding and documentation: Do our physicians and mid-level providers code and document effectively for both clinical and billing purposes?
- Receivables management: Is our revenue cycle management engine operating at peak capacity?
- Service mix: Do we offer the cognitive, procedural, and ancillary services our patients and their referring physicians expect to find in our medical practices?

This discussion is further amplified in chapter 8.

Tenet 3: Of the eight revenue factors, physician productivity is the major driver of medical practice revenue. The major driver of physician productivity, in turn, is a performance-based compensation model that places a significant amount (30–50 percent) of an established physician's compensation at risk on a monthly basis (see chapter 7). A secondary driver of physician productivity is an effective clinical assistant who recognizes that his or her most important role is to support high-quality care and caring, followed by managing the physician's productivity. Highest and best-use staffing principles are discussed in chapter 8.

Tenet 4: Quality care is good business; it is not an excuse for poor productivity. Medical professionals are trained to provide quality medical services. They are licensed and credentialed to provide quality care. They should not be practicing if they fail to do so. For this reason, performance pay priorities should be volume and customer service related, both of which drive practice performance. Those who fail to meet quality standards should not be employed in this profession.

Tenet 5: The health care decision maker for the family is usually the woman. She typically selects a primary care provider for her family whose location is within a reasonable distance of home and the children's schools. (She will drive further for her own care.) She forms a long-term relationship with "the doctor," who is usually a family physician, general internist, or pediatrician, and she forms a relationship with an obstetrician/gynecologist for her own care. She is almost totally dependent on her trusted primary care providers for referrals to specialists (e.g., to determine both when a referral is necessary and which specialist to see).

Tenet 6: Given the unique cost structure of medical practices (largely dominated by the cost of human resources), relatively few traditional economies of scale are available to exploit. Cramming multiple physicians in a big-box structure in the name of scale economies is not a useful strategy (although a few legitimate reasons support the need for a big-box office space). Patients do prefer a convenient, one-stop shop but despise big, confusing facilities with huge parking garages. They prefer a well-equipped primary care location convenient to home. This preference argues for smaller primary care practices geared toward capturing and retaining market share within a five-mile radius, supplemented by an occasional big-box space with specialists and more complex ancillary services "so I don't have to drive all the way to the hospital."

Tenet 7: If established physicians are losing money in private practice, hospital acquisition will not fix the problem. Purchase only practices that are financially and operationally viable. Acquiring one dysfunctional practice can consume many times its value in management time and attention.

Tenet 8: Primary care equals market share for employed and affiliated specialty physicians, as well as for the hospital. Having plenty of viable primary care practices is the foundation of a successful network and a sustainable competitive advantage.

Tenet 9: Noting that some hospital executives want their physician organizations to be perceived as physician led, ***physicians must be engaged as partners with senior hospital executives for the integrated model to work.*** Indeed, there is great power in engaging physicians to lead hospital-owned medical practice networks. But the hospital CEO is the board-appointed fiduciary and should not abdicate that responsibility, particularly with primary care physicians who hold the hospital's market share and/or direct it to the hospital in the form of referrals. Physician expertise and perspective should be included in the operational governance of medical practice networks through the council model rather than being used for implementation management. Hence, successful hospital-owned physician networks are *partnership led.* The council model discussed in chapter 3 facilitates that engagement.

Tenet 10: Management is implementation. People with medical degrees are not necessarily good managers (although some are excellent managers, with or without an MBA). For this reason, multiple medical directors and multiple physician/management dyads do not usually work in a practice setting. Networks and the individual groups that comprise them need good managers. Build a management team around good leaders, with or without medical degrees, and implementation will be successful. (Good leaders without medical degrees usually cost less to employ than those with degrees. The highest and best use of physician expertise is usually in the examination room, procedure room, or operating room.)

Structuring the Hospital-Owned Network

A great temptation may arise to call in the attorneys and draw a "new box" on the organizational chart before completing the operating plan. But heeding that temptation violates the fundamental management principle that "form follows function." Substituting a revised legal organization structure for good planning may be expedient, but it is never recommended. Properly defining the medical practice network vision and operational functions informs structural decisions. No operating plan is complete, however, without the appropriate legal structure to facilitate its implementation.

Over the years, we have seen a variety of legal models, many of which have been successful. Some have structured the hospital-owned medical practice network as a for-profit subsidiary of the hospital. Others have been organized as wholly owned, not-for-profit subsidiaries. Some organizations have chosen to employ the physicians under the hospital umbrella and the support staff and billing services under a separate network organization, often called a management services organization (MSO).

Some organizations keep the network assets in the hospital legal entity and lease them to the MSO. Others hold the practice assets in one organization and buy MSO services from another. The organization should be structured according to the advice of legal counsel. In addition to the operating plan, the organization's current legal structure, its tax status, the flow of capital, and its strategic plan will influence the ultimate design.

On a separate but very important note, where multiple affiliated hospitals form a local system (e.g., same large metropolitan area), we *do not recommend* the establishment of a physician network and network infrastructure for each hospital. Instead, we recommend that the network be organized at the local system level to manage the primary care and specialty practices of all physicians employed by that system. This structure has proven to be the most effective at ensuring high-quality care, consistent customer service, improved physician productivity, and increased financial viability. The network executive works closely with each hospital executive to ensure that system-owned primary care and specialty practices fulfill their part of local hospital strategy.

Summary

A properly structured operating plan helps those involved in the process to understand the "theory of the business" of medical practice network management and how it differs from hospital management. It is a reminder of the integrated vision for the medical practice network and documents its purpose as part of organizational memory. An operating plan is a reminder of the commitment to applying correct principles when a sense of expediency triggered by a money-losing physician or a dysfunctional practice is tempting to heed. An operating plan establishes performance expectations for anyone who chooses to join the network. It provides guidelines for both operational governance and the management/implementation team.

References

1. P. Drucker, *Peter Drucker on the Profession of Management,* 22 (Boston: Harvard Business School Publishing, 1998).
2. Ibid., 123.
3. Ibid., 123.
4. Ibid., 124.
5. Daryl R. Conner, *Managing at the Speed of Change,* 116 (New York: Villard Books, 1992).
6. M. Halley, P. Holtman, and A. Shaffer, "Physician Integration Economics" [http://www.halleyconsulting.com/tasks/sites/hcg/assets/File/Physician_Integration_ Economics_07082009.pdf]. Accessed July 13, 2010.
7. M. Halley and R. Lloyd, "How to Break Even on an Acquired Primary Care Network," *Healthcare Financial Management* (November 2000): 69–74.

CHAPTER 3

Engaging Physicians in Operational Governance

The term *governance* is usually associated with boards of trustees or directors. These groups are formed to oversee the success of ventures large and small. They are often composed of seasoned executives or content experts who contribute their wisdom and knowledge to senior leadership. A board frequently holds the chief executive officer (CEO) accountable for proposing and implementing strategies that will ensure both short- and long-term viability for the organization.

Boards participate in strategy development and approve major tactics and policies designed to implement that strategy. Board members oversee financial performance, manage executive compensation, approve capital and operating budgets, and are increasingly held accountable to oversee compliance with laws and regulations. Board members have a formal fiduciary responsibility as part of their oversight role.

Operational Governance

For our purposes, *operational governance* shares many characteristics with fiduciary boards. However, most operational governance models do not have formal authority in the traditional board sense (although some are formed with board approval). They derive their authority from an officer of the organization, usually the hospital CEO, who participates as a member and who has ultimate veto authority. Operational governing bodies are subject to the same board-approved strategies and policies as every other council, committee, or department of the organization.

Operational governance does include responsibility for ensuring the development of strategies in support of the larger organization's mission, strategy, and performance objectives. It also includes the development of performance standards, establishment of performance improvement initiatives, and review of financial and operating performance throughout a medical practice network. This type of governance holds a management team accountable for implementing both network-wide and site-specific policies, tactics, and initiatives.

Operational governance involves the approval of operating policies and procedures affecting the business and clinical sides of affiliated practices. It also includes recommendations to the board-appointed fiduciary and/or board on such issues as budget and physician compensation. The operational governing body cannot hire, fire, or sanction employed physicians, although members will review performance and make recommendations to the CEO, who signs the employment contracts.

The Council Model

Operational governance is best provided through a council model. A true council model is not a rubber-stamp organization or an information-disseminating vehicle. A council combines the expertise of knowledge workers (e.g., clinical expertise, financial expertise, operating expertise) with the line management authority of the CEO and others to ensure the success of the network. Council members provide line managers with counsel based on their content expertise, which usually results in improved group decision making. A full-time practicing physician typically chairs the council and works with the hospital CEO on the business of the council.

Because council members participate in the decision-making process, they are in an ideal position to become what Daryl Conner calls "sustaining sponsors,"[1] as the CEO and other implementers manage change within their areas of responsibility. Because physician leaders participate in the decision-making process, they understand the factors that affect important decisions and they are more likely to take ownership of those decisions.

While physicians cannot be supervised in the traditional sense, they can be effectively held accountable by a CEO with the advice of the council's experts, who are also physicians. For example, it is not uncommon for a physician with behavioral problems to receive a visit from both the CEO, who signs his employment contract, and the chairperson of the operations governance council, who is a full-time practicing physician. This combination of clinical expertise and "legal" authority sets the stage for the types of crucial conversations (discussed in more detail later) that are sometimes necessary in such sessions.[2]

Some physicians, bitter from past experience, have rejected the council model as simply another political vehicle for management to use in influencing physician leaders' peers by virtue of their medical degrees. Traditional advisory boards that have no influence in decision making are not councils. Properly functioning councils are forums to engage the key decision maker—the CEO—in principle-based decisions. In a well-functioning council, the CEO participates as a member of the body. Its physician and executive members discuss issues, approve policies, receive reports, and make decisions with the participation of the board-appointed fiduciary—again, the CEO.

Only rarely does a CEO exercise veto authority. This authority is used for two reasons: First, and foremost, physician leaders realize they must make decisions based on correct principles; otherwise, the CEO will be forced to use his or her veto. Second, wise CEOs understand the value of the operations council forum and will not violate the trust that naturally develops as members work together and with the CEO to identify and implement correct principles.

The CEO also participates in the discussions about important issues, making sure that decisions are principle based. CEOs who have been members of properly functioning operations councils indicate that after the first few meetings, as council members become comfortable with one another, they hold each other accountable for making good decisions. At that point, the CEOs rarely need to redirect discussions.

The Network Operations Council

A vital component of successful medical practice network ownership is the network operations council (NOC). The NOC is usually composed of six employed physicians and three hospital executives, one of whom is the hospital CEO. The CEO should select an employed physician to serve as NOC chairperson and as one of the six clinical council members. She should consider the NOC chairperson choice as carefully as she would any other senior executive selection. The chairperson and the CEO are then responsible to select or ensure the selection of the other five physician members, who are chosen primarily for their leadership ability. Other selection criteria may include specialty representation, geographic representation, practice experience, and leadership development.

The NOC is not a representative government, and physician members should not be selected by popular vote. The physician members of the NOC will likely serve staggered terms to allow more physician involvement and leadership development over time.

The NOC physician chairperson sets the tone for the NOC and for the network. His or her influence will be felt first by other members of the NOC, then by chartered subcommittees, and ultimately by each physician and other provider who participates in a practice operations council (POC). Appendix A is an example of a role description for the NOC physician chairperson.

Ideally, the NOC chairperson is a well-respected primary care physician with an exemplary practice, great communications skills, leadership experience, and the motivation to influence his or her peers to tackle even the toughest challenges.

In addition to the hospital CEO, the executive members of the NOC usually include the hospital chief financial officer and one other executive. These three serve ex officio and are responsible for learning the theory of success in the medical practice network business so they can properly partner with physician leaders and contribute to that success. As the board-appointed fiduciary, the hospital CEO authorizes and legitimizes the NOC and its decisions. As the legal authority or officer, the CEO signs the physician employment agreements. He or she must also ultimately approve (or veto) NOC decisions. The physician practice network executive should not serve as a member of the NOC for reasons discussed in chapter 4.

The primary purposes of the NOC are the following:

1. Engage the employed physicians and mid-level providers as partners with senior management in sponsoring, or championing, the success of the physician network in support of an integrated strategy.
2. Identify and implement correct operating principles for the network as a whole and for each hospital-owned medical practice.
3. Engage employed physicians and senior management in support of the four critical success filters. Monitor the progress of each practice and physician toward achieving those performance targets within a specified timeline.
4. Support the establishment of clinical and service quality measurement and initiatives within the clinics, including accreditation or licensure requirements.
5. Hold the network executive and other members of the management team and billing office accountable for the revenue cycle management process and outcomes.
6. Hold the network executive accountable to develop the infrastructure and implement network-wide and site-specific initiatives that will facilitate practices achieving their performance targets.
7. Hold individual employed physicians and mid-level providers accountable for achieving private practice levels of performance in order to support the implementation of NOC-approved policies in individual practice settings and to fulfill their contractual obligations.
8. Ensure that *every willing provider* has the opportunity to be successful. (The NOC annually reviews and recommends to the CEO the continuation of each employed provider's contractual relationship.)
9. Provide feedback to the payer negotiating team on proposed payer contracts and terms. At least quarterly, the NOC should invite the payer negotiator to the NOC meeting to discuss payer performance.
10. Approve *all operating and billing policies* affecting the practices.

As the network evolves, and as legitimate tasks arise to be performed, it is recommended that subcommittees of the NOC be established to work on behalf of the council. Each subcommittee is chaired by a physician member of the NOC and includes other employed physicians with an interest in the subcommittee charter. The subcommittee chairperson represents the committee at NOC meetings and ensures that the subcommittee abides by its charter. Subcommittees chartered by an NOC might include the following:

1. *Quality assurance.* Proposes standards, sponsors performance improvement initiatives, and monitors performance in clinical quality and service quality.
2. *Operations.* Monitors operational performance, including the billing office and revenue cycle process. Supports the network executive in establishing operating policies for recommendation to the NOC.
3. *Compensation.* Accepts responsibility for developing or adopting and recommending a compensation model for physicians and other providers. Also monitors physician performance under the approved model to ensure that physicians who are willing to work can and do earn market-competitive compensation.
4. *Specialty services.* Works to develop and maintain relationships between employed specialists of choice[3] and referring physicians and facilitates relationships with ancillary providers within the network and the hospital.

Again, as subcommittees are established, physicians or mid-level providers who are not members of the NOC should staff them in order to engage more providers in operational governance activity.

In markets where multiple affiliated hospitals form a local system (e.g., single large metropolitan area), the challenge of operational governance becomes more complex, although the fundamental principles remain intact. As mentioned in chapter 2, we recommend that the local system form only one medical practice network organization to employ all physicians for all local system hospitals. Operational governance of these practices should still include six employed physicians, one of whom is the chairperson. The executive members may vary. We recommend that the senior executive be the individual who signs the physician employment contracts. Further, we recommend that the senior executive report to the local system CEO, as would each local hospital CEO. We also recommend that the NOC include a senior financial officer and a local system–level executive. The system CEO should be invited to attend the NOC as often as possible.

Practice Operations Councils

The network operations council focuses on network-wide initiatives that affect all practices in the organization. Those initiatives, such as physician compensation models and revenue cycle management policies, can contribute significantly to operational performance improvement. But no network ever achieved success through network-wide initiatives alone. Without performance improvement at each practice, specific to that site, performance improvement efforts fall short of their potential. As with network-wide initiatives, success at the site level requires effective operational governance at each practice and implementation of site-specific initiatives by competent management.

Practice-level operational governance is provided by a practice operations council at each location. The POC is composed of all physicians and other providers in the practice. It also includes the network executive or his or her designee, that is, the line officer to whom the practice manager reports. The practice manager is not a member of the POC but is accountable to the POC and the line manager. The POC meets monthly and has the following responsibilities:

1. Ensures that the practice achieves its clinical quality, service quality, provider productivity, and financial performance targets and timelines
2. Ensures the success of every willing provider in the practice
3. Sponsors NOC policies to ensure their proper implementation at the practice site
4. Holds the practice manager accountable to implement under the direction of the POC
5. Provides input to the NOC
6. Ensures that the practice has the right support staff, processes, training, and equipment to operate successfully and within the context of the critical success filters
7. Ensures performance improvement at the practice site

Practice operations councils are usually small in size and do not have a formal leader (although the practice manager or network executive will often facilitate the meetings). The practice manager provides an agenda to which all POC members contribute, and he or she keeps minutes of past meetings and decisions. Council members depend on effective dialogue skills (discussed later in this chapter) to address issues with each other and barriers to performance. Issues that cannot be resolved by the POC are transferred by the executive POC member to the NOC for resolution.

A typical POC meets monthly to review clinical and service quality results, provider performance, and financial outcomes. Each POC works with its practice manager to develop revenue enhancement, expense control, and other performance improvement initiatives, which are documented in a site-specific action plan (see Appendix B). Revenue and expense tactics are assigned to project leaders along with a due date and estimated performance impact. The POC sponsors those initiatives and holds the practice manager accountable to effectively implement approved tactics. The POC also carefully monitors the performance impact to make sure that successfully implemented tactics achieve the anticipated results. Successes are celebrated in staff meetings, and failed tactics are supplemented by modified or additional initiatives to achieve the desired overall results.

Characteristics of Successful Councils

When we coach new NOCs, we start with the premise that groups can make better decisions than individuals can, especially when dealing with complex problems or issues requiring creative solutions. James Surowiecki, author of *The Wisdom of Crowds,* wrote: "Under the right circumstances, groups are remarkably intelligent, and are often smarter than the smartest people in them."[4] In our experience, councils composed of primary care physicians, specialty physicians, and hospital executives can indeed be "remarkably intelligent" and can solve even the most complex issues as they overcome we/they barriers and learn to think and work as a unit for the benefit of all. Such capability involves a willingness on the part of hospital CEOs to truly *engage* physicians—and their points of view—as *partners* in the success of the enterprise. Similarly, it involves willingness on the part of physicians to be good business partners and to make good business decisions demonstrating the same passion with which they make good clinical decisions—recognizing that both are critical.

Effective council models start with a great NOC, one that has the following characteristics:

- The right leader
- The right members
- Commitment to fundamental tenets
- A shared vision
- Effective sponsorship
- A culture of accountability

The Right Leader

A highly functioning NOC requires a successful physician leader to partner with the hospital CEO in establishing the council model. We have already discussed the role of the NOC chairperson. The selection of that physician leader should be made as carefully as the selection of any leader within the integrated delivery system. Leadership skills are the first prerequisite. Outstanding clinical experience and productivity are also vitally important, as is having the respect of physician peers.

The Right Members

The physician chairperson must be joined by several other physician leaders with similar characteristics. These leaders are usually selected by the hospital CEO and the physician chairperson. The right members are committed to governing well, to understanding the factors critical to the success of the hospital-owned medical practice network and its individual practices, and to effectively implementing those principles.

Commitment to Fundamental Tenets

Successful NOC members develop and adhere to certain fundamental tenets as the foundation of their council meetings and subcommittee meetings. These tenets include the development of "principled policies," that is, policies and procedures based on correct operating principles. They are committed to the four critical success filters in making every decision and in approving every policy, procedure, strategy, and tactic. Recall that those filters include the following:

- The initiative maintains or enhances clinical quality as defined by our physicians.
- The initiative maintains or enhances service quality as defined by our patients and their referring physicians.
- The initiative maintains or enhances physician productivity.
- The initiative maintains or enhances practice operational and financial viability.

Council members are committed to rigorously measuring the organization's performance in all four areas. They insist on sharing timely and accurate information, making it transparent throughout the organization. They make decisions based on fact as the currency of effective decision making and performance management. They learn from experience, both positive and negative.

A Shared Vision

Network operations council members acknowledge the network's role in supporting the integrated system mission and vision. They develop a vision for the network in support of the overall strategy. Council members do not simply adopt the hospital's mission, because the network is not a hospital. Nor do they adopt a practice vision that is devoid of hospital strategy. Instead, they create a compelling vision that represents the synergy available in linking employed primary care providers with specialty services (employed or otherwise), hospital service lines, and ancillaries in an integrated delivery system. It is a vision that defines the network's role in capturing and retaining market share and referring that market share when specialty and hospital services are indicated.

Effective Sponsorship

Daryl Conner defines sponsors as those who approve initiatives, set priorities, and provide reinforcement during implementation.[5] The initiating sponsor is the CEO, described in chapter 1 as the market manager, who is the buck stop for the organization. Other members of the NOC and the POCs become sustaining sponsors, who support implementation of approved initiatives at the network and practice levels. Although managers are the implementers, councils support and reinforce that implementation. Importantly, as a fundamental tenet, council members commit to supporting council decisions, both publicly and privately. Although some policies or initiatives may come down to a majority vote, all NOC and POC members support the outcome.

A Culture of Accountability

A key difference between successful long-term organizations and those that fail to develop a sustainable strategy is that successful organizations develop a culture of accountability.[6] For our purposes, a culture of accountability includes clear performance targets and timelines, effective delegation of responsibility for achieving those targets within the timelines, rigorous measurement of performance, a commitment to finishing the job, and a willingness to remove those (physicians, management, and others) who fail to deliver the desired results or who violate fundamental tenets.

Importantly, knowledge of proper council procedures is only part of the process of developing an effective network operations council and practice operations councils. Success also requires experience and practice as individual members and as a council.

The Practice of Dialogue

One of the most important skills for a successful council model is the ability of council members to dialogue effectively. Dialogue allows council members to engage one another in the success of the practice and the network. Dialogue is the ability to openly and respectfully address issues where differing personal views, motives, and agendas may be present. Effective dialogue includes the willingness of council members to subordinate "who is right" to "what is right" for the practice, their patients, referring physicians, and the support staff.

When we teach our clients about effective dialogue, we use two important books as resources. The first is *The Fifth Discipline*, by Peter Senge.[7] The second is *Crucial Conversations: Tools for Talking When the Stakes Are High*, by Kerry Patterson and colleagues.[8]

Peter Senge teaches us that effective dialogue helps council members:

- Reach beyond their individual understanding by actively listening to the perspectives and experience of others
- Hold their points of view "gently," being open to the influence of others, whose suggestions are often insightful based on their unique experience
- Help each other broaden their thinking by openly sharing their opinions and encouraging others to do the same

- Encourage people to share their full experience and assumptions about an issue
- Take advantage of seeing difficult issues from many points of view, opening themselves to new solutions and possibilities
- Communicate their assumptions freely to others but suspend them long enough to learn from others
- Make it safe to become observers of their own thinking
- Remain collegial rather than adversarial

The authors of *Crucial Conversations* define *dialogue* as "the free flow of meaning between two or more people."[9] Their comprehensive treatise defines a crucial conversation as one in which the stakes are high (high risk), emotions run strong, and sharply opposing viewpoints are at play.[10] The following are a few helpful highlights for council members from *Crucial Conversations*:

- *Silence or violence.* The authors indicate that when crucial topics arise in meetings or in conversation, people move to "violence" or to "silence." We have all been in meetings where one player dominates the conversation, pressing his opinion and discounting or discrediting all others. "Only an idiot would see things differently" is his unsubtle message. The rest of us, not wanting to look like idiots, sit back, fold our arms, and remain quiet—we move to silence. This scenario is detrimental to establishing "a free flow of meaning" or "what is right." Agenda items appear again, over time, as they remain unresolved.
- *Build safety.* The authors discuss the importance of creating a safe environment in which violence is not tolerated and all points of view are solicited to create and expand the "pool of available meaning." Establishing dialogue as a fundamental tenet and protecting it is the responsibility of every council member, particularly the chairperson.
- *Individual commitment.* Council members are encouraged to improve dialogue by starting with the only person they can influence—themselves. We are encouraged to become aware of our biases and perceptions, as well as their influence on our responses during crucial conversations. We are counseled to develop listening skills and to respectfully engage one another.
- *Kinder and gentler.* The authors dispute the idea that being open, honest, or direct (or even brilliant) without being respectful of others is acceptable behavior. They insist—and we agree—that being *both* direct *and* respectful is the only acceptable operating model in a council setting. Expressing opinions while respecting the differing opinions of others adds to that pool of information available to council members for effective decision making.

Sponsorship versus Implementation

In the next chapter, we discuss the development of a management or implementation team. Before doing so, here we distinguish between the roles of operational governance and management. Table 3-1 highlights those differences.

Operations councils must take care not to become involved in managing the implementation process. Likewise, managers cannot be sponsors. Failure to recognize these distinct roles produces frustration and yields short tenure for management.

Summary

Keeping employed physicians engaged with line management is critical to the success and sustainability of every hospital-owned medical practice network. An effective operational governance model ensures that these medical practice networks are *partnership led*. The council model recommends that operational governance occur for the network as a whole and for each medical practice that is part of the network. Every physician and mid-level provider is engaged in operational governance at one of these two levels. Line management validates the authority of these councils, and line managers are accountable to them as implementers. Effective dialogue is the cultural standard for these operational governing bodies to the benefit of the organization; physicians; support staff; and, most importantly, those they serve.

Table 3-1. Roles of Operational Governance and of Management

Issue	Operations Council	Management
Vision	Develops vision for the network and individual practices (where appropriate)	Implements the vision of the sponsors
Strategy and Tactics	Approves and sponsors strategy and tactics	Suggests strategy and develops tactics for approval based on correct principles
Sponsorship	Prioritizes and determines the pace of implementation; provides reinforcement as needed	Implements and reports implementation progress to councils
Performance Expectations	Establishes performance expectations	Measures and reports performance to NOC and POCs
Policy and Procedures	Approves policies and procedures	Suggests policies and procedures based on correct principles and implements approved policies and procedures
Accountability	Holds physicians, mid-level providers, and management accountable for behaviors and results	Holds support staff accountable for behaviors and results

References

1. Daryl R. Conner, *Managing and the Speed of Change,* 116 (New York: Villard, 1992).
2. Kerry Patterson, Joseph Grenny, Ron McMillan, and Al Switzler, *Crucial Conversations: Tools for Talking When the Stakes Are High* (New York: McGraw-Hill, 2002).
3. K. Cohn and D. Hough, eds., *Practice Management,* 48–50, vol. 1, *The Business of Healthcare* (Westport, CT: Praeger, 2008).
4. J. Surowiecki, *The Wisdom of Crowds,* xiii (New York: Doubleday, 2004).
5. Conner, *Managing and the Speed of Change,* 116.
6. M. Halley, "A Culture of Accountability: What Distinguishes an Exceptional Medical Group," *Group Practice Journal* 54, no. 3 (2005): 10–14.
7. P. Senge, *The Fifth Discipline* (New York: Doubleday, 1990).
8. Patterson et al., *Crucial Conversations.*
9. Ibid., 20.
10. Ibid., 3.

CHAPTER 4

Management Infrastructure

A common problem in hospital-owned medical practices is confusion over who is the boss. Now that the physicians are on the payroll, do they report to the office manager, like other employees? Do they report to the network executive? Do the nurses report to the doctors or to the office manager? Who holds whom accountable?

We have already discussed the fact that physicians, as knowledge workers, cannot be supervised in the traditional sense but must still be held accountable. Clinical support staff members are certainly accountable to the physicians to whom they are assigned in clinical matters, but what about when issues of office policy and process arise?

Who's the Boss?

Best practice experience has demonstrated that operations governance through a council model clarifies these physician accountability questions. Recall that the practice operations council (POC) consists of all providers in the practice plus the network executive or designee. Physicians are accountable to each other within a properly functioning POC, as they would be in a private office setting.

Some issues may arise, however, that cannot be resolved at the POC level. They are elevated by the network executive to the network operations council (NOC), where the hospital chief executive officer (CEO), who signs the physician employment agreements, has the legal authority to hold these contract employees accountable to meet expectations. The CEO and the physician NOC chairperson, in counsel with other NOC members as needed, meet with the occasional aberrant physician to clarify policy, discuss behavior, or terminate contractual relationships.

Best practice management structure conforms to the operational governance model at the network and site levels, as illustrated in figure 4-1. The network operations council holds the network executive accountable to implement network-wide initiatives. Each POC (which includes the network executive or designee among its members) holds its assigned practice manager accountable to implement policies and procedures approved by the local council. The practice manager then holds all support staff accountable to follow those policies and procedures. In short, the POC is the boss of the practice manager who is the boss of the support staff, including nurses. Under the direction of the POC, the practice manager and support staff are accountable to assist *every willing physician* to be successful in the practice setting.

Figure 4-1. Operational Governance and Management Structure

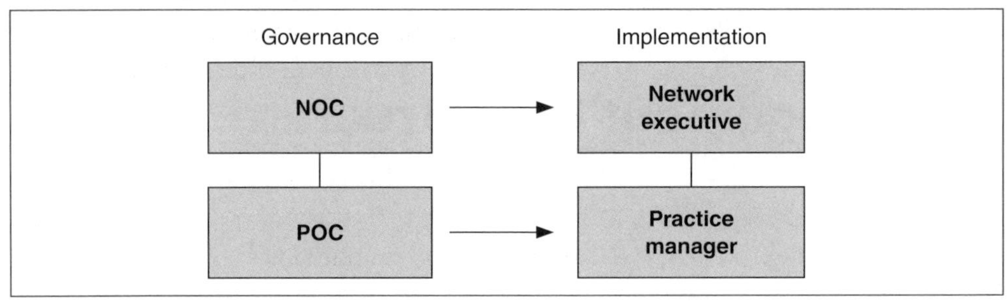

Note: NOC = network operations council; POC = practice operations council.
Source: Halley Consulting Group. www.halleyconsulting.com.

Managers in a council setting are *implementers* who do the bidding of the councils and who manage support staff to help physicians and other providers deliver high-quality clinical care and top-quality customer service effectively and efficiently (high productivity yields financial viability). Managers do not act without the sponsorship of their respective councils.

Management as Implementer

As discussed in chapter 3, operations councils are more than advisory boards or figurehead groups. Network operations councils set direction in support of the integrated delivery system strategies; they establish performance standards, set policies, review performance, and hold physicians and managers accountable for successful implementation.

Again, the network executive is responsible for ensuring the effective implementation of network-wide initiatives approved by the NOC and communicated to all physicians through the NOC meeting minutes. Such initiatives include policies and procedures that affect every practice (or at least multiple practices) in the network. For example, most networks have standard policies for revenue cycle management and to govern human resource issues. Similarly, software decisions involving practice management and medical records are usually network-wide initiatives. Network development strategies, capital allocation, and quality assurance are also common NOC matters.

A critical role of the network executive is to ensure that every practice location is assigned a competent practice manager. Small group practice managers are rarely master's degree prepared or even college trained. In fact, many start out as medical practice receptionists and simply stay at the practice longer than anyone else. They are often very bright daily operations experts who have learned management on the job. These small-practice managers are like sponges when given the opportunity to learn the theories and principles of professional management. They need to be provided with tools, taught correct principles, and coached in their implementation to become management professionals; the tools, training, and coaching are provided at the network level. Such support ensures that practice managers are prepared to work with physicians and other providers in POCs to successfully implement site-specific initiatives.

As implementers, the management team (executives and managers) works for the councils and supervises support staff (both clinical and nonclinical) to achieve the organization's objectives as defined by the councils. The physicians and other providers are accountable to those same councils.

Authorizing Managers

Line management authority in a best practice network setting starts with the hospital CEO, who is the board-appointed fiduciary and market manager. That authority is delegated by the CEO to a network executive who, in turn, delegates authority to several practice managers to act on behalf of the organization. These three levels of management provide the most efficient use of authority and streamlined accountability. However, depending on the size and complexity of the integrated delivery organization and the medical practice network, this model may need to be modified. Larger physician networks usually require the addition of directors between the network executive and practice manager levels. Each director is accountable for eight to ten practice locations.

In addition, and as a last resort, the hospital CEO may need to delegate authority to another senior executive to supervise the network executive. This five-layer model is not nearly as efficient as the three-level model, but it may be necessary as a medical practice network grows. Each of the five management roles is described below.

Market Manager

As discussed in chapter 1, today's hospital CEOs must manage well beyond the boundaries of the hospital campus. They must be *market* managers who understand how to capture market share in targeted neighborhoods through the proper placement of or affiliation with primary care practices. They understand the importance of employing or affiliating with specialists of choice to attract referrals from those primary care physicians (PCPs) who hold that market share. They also understand the importance of integrating these top-quality specialists with strategic service lines to offer the best service delivery and outcomes. As strategists, market managers must appropriately invest capital to ensure that all components of the integrated system function properly to meet the needs, wants, and priorities of patients and referring physicians, who are all part of the "demand chain."[1] A demand chain is a partnership linking the hospital-based specialists with relevant hospital departments, specialty physicians, and PCPs (discussed more fully in chapter 5).

In addition to allocating capital to support an integration strategy, the market manager must facilitate the development and maintenance of appropriate referral relationships among physicians and between physicians and the hospital. Regulations and laws restrict these relationships from being based on incentives or kickbacks of any kind. Referring physician relationships must instead be based on factors such as ease of access to the specialist, the hospital, and ancillary services; trust that the specialist and the hospital will provide high-quality care and caring to patients referred; timely feedback to the referring provider; and the opportunity for the PCP to participate in coordinating the patient's care and follow-up. Relationships and service levels should be the market manager's priorities. And just as important, the CEO–market manager must exercise the line authority to ensure that service barriers (including inadequate policies, procedures, facilities, equipment, managers, and staff) are eliminated and that service failures are analyzed and corrected.

For these reasons, the hospital CEO–market manager should personally participate with his or her physician partners as a member of the NOC. Ideally, the medical practice network executive would report directly to the hospital CEO to ensure that the CEO–market manager remains attuned to the performance issues associated with these critical employed physician partners.

Increasingly, hospitals and health systems realize the vital role of market managers as strategic integrators.[2] Some health systems are changing their performance measurement dashboards to include a broader range of indicators for each local market. These organizations are unwilling to tolerate substandard hospital-owned medical practice performance that is masked by a hospital's bottom line.

Health system leaders expect employed physicians to perform at the same high level as their private practice counterparts. They expect their market managers to understand and implement the principles of successful medical practice network management to the same degree that they understand and implement the principles of successful hospital management. They expect capital allocations to yield more than the latest technology surrounded by bricks and mortar. Enlightened system leaders expect their market managers to use a portion of their capital to support a primary care retail strategy to capture the market share that will guarantee the long-term viability of the hospital and its affiliated specialists. They expect their market managers to manage relationships and performance all along the demand chain to attract and retain that market share instead of seeing it bleed to competitors.

A successful market manager is, first and foremost, a strategist with a keen understanding of physician integration economics. He acknowledges and understands the unique critical success factors driving each business line in an integrated system. He is a superb relationship manager who understands that successful relationships must reach beyond an employment contract or a common payroll.

He has the personality and the skill to naturally implement what Theodore Levitt defined as factors—positive and negative—that affect successful long-term relationships.[3] Those factors are listed in table 4-1.

The role of the market manager defines the ideal candidate. He must be a strategist with an understanding of market dynamics and physician integration. He must possess the ability to comfortably dialogue with physicians and engage them as partners (both employed and otherwise) in pursuit of market strategy. The candidate must have unquestioned integrity among physicians, executives, and support staff. Fairness is a key attribute. He must also have credibility that is based on past experience, past relationships, and prior decisions. The ideal candidate will have the ability to balance short-term performance with sustainable, long-term strategies both within and outside the hospital. Having the right market manager sponsoring the initiative over time is the key to a successful physician integration strategy.

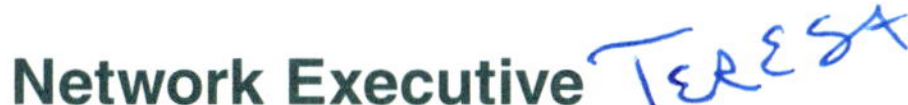

Network Executive

The role of the network executive and the experience required are functions of current medical practice network size and projected growth. However, the knowledge and ability needed by a successful network executive are the same regardless

Table 4-1. Factors Affecting Successful Long-Term Relationships

Positive Factors	Negative Factors
Initiate positive phone calls	Make only callbacks
Make recommendations	Make justifications
Candor in language	Accommodative language
Use phone	Use correspondence
Show appreciation	Wait for misunderstandings
Make service suggestions	Wait for service requests
Use "we" problem-solving language	Use "owe us" legal language
Get to problems	Respond to problems
Use jargon/shorthand	Use long-winded communications
Air personality problems	Hide personality problems
Talk of "our future together"	Talk of making good on the past
Make responses routine	Respond in fire drill/emergency mode
Accept responsibility	Shift blame
Plan the future	Rehash the past

of network size. The ideal candidate needs a thorough knowledge of medical practice business operations, including the policies and processes that support all twelve critical success factors and the four critical success filters defined earlier in the book.[4]

The network executive needs to understand the anatomy of an office visit, how to effectively provide ancillary services, and how to accommodate ambulatory procedures. She also needs to understand the fundamentals of a successful surgery practice and how to balance evaluation and surgical activity. In addition, the network executive must understand how to implement highest and best-use staffing to ensure efficiency in medical practice settings.[5] A thorough knowledge of financial and statistical data and the proper evaluation of that information are essential for a network executive.

The most critical ability of the ideal network executive is effective communication. The leader must possess both verbal and written communication skills and be an effective listener. The network executive must also possess the ability to hold crucial conversations, meaning the ability to facilitate conversations "where (1) the stakes are high, (2) opinions vary, and (3) emotions run strong."[6] This skill will need to be combined with the ability to effectively manage organizational change, including soliciting sponsorship from the CEO and other members of operations councils.

The successful network executive will understand how to manage initiatives and performance in a setting that features at least one distinct culture for each practice, including the hospital and health system cultures in which the network is nested. The successful network executive will be an effective coach and a teacher of correct principles and their proper implementation. He will understand how to effectively delegate responsibility and authority. Importantly, the network executive will have the ability to hold management and support staff accountable for both process and outcomes.

Smaller networks, those constituting fewer than ten locations and twenty-five physicians, require an operations expert to serve as a hands-on coach. Network executives functioning in these settings will need to deal with network-wide issues and to coach for site-specific performance. They will facilitate the NOC, implementing appropriate network-wide initiatives such as revenue cycle management policies and software adoption, with each POC.

Small-network executives will spend most of their time working with each POC and each practice manager to develop site-specific action plans (see Appendix B) that drive performance improvement at each practice location. The coaching process requires weekly interaction and involvement by the network executive in each practice. Consequently, the network executive in these settings can only manage eight to ten locations, depending on their proximity to each other, the capabilities of practice managers, and the complexity of medical practice issues. The ideal small-network executive will have several years of experience as a practice manager; a master's degree in business, public health, or health care administration; and multi-site management experience.

Larger networks require a network executive with the operational experience and abilities identified earlier. Importantly, the qualified leader will have executive-level experience and a proven track record of performance in the following areas:

- Management of large, multi-site, multispecialty networks
- Engagement of physicians in the development and implementation of competitive strategies in support of the integrated delivery system
- Direction of multiple management levels for results
- Successful facilitation of a governing body with multiple subcommittees
- Network development through large practice acquisition and physician employment contracting
- Successful development and management of leaders to achieve performance objectives across multiple locations
- Direction of others in successfully implementing significant network-wide initiatives (e.g., electronic medical records software selection and implementation)
- Hospital and/or health system executive experience and interaction with senior executives/strategists
- Effective management of staff specialists to include human resources, quality assurance, finance and accounting, revenue cycle management, and other areas likely to report directly to her in a large network

This seasoned executive will spend most of her time facilitating the NOC and managing directors who manage practice managers. The network executive will deal with network-wide performance improvement, including supporting NOC subcommittees for quality, physician compensation, operations (including revenue cycle), and financial performance. She will formulate network-wide policies for consideration and approval by the NOC and its subcommittees; provide financial oversight of and direct resources to struggling practices; help formulate and implement network strategy in support of hospital strategic objectives to capture market share and attract that market share to selected service lines; and create a culture of accountability among managers and support staff and facilitate that culture for physicians using the NOC. She will be personally accountable to the CEO and the NOC. This executive will likely possess a master's degree and have at least ten years of relevant experience.

Practice Manager

While some medical practice networks include large group practices, most are a collection of formerly independent smaller offices ranging in size from one to six providers. As mentioned earlier, unlike hospital departments, in which many managers have extensive management training and college degrees, most small medical office managers are daily operations experts who have not received much formal management training. Private practice office managers have been expected to implement the physicians' wishes while keeping the physicians' world stable and predictable. Some small group practice managers have never seen a practice financial statement; many are not held accountable to manage to the bottom line. Solo and small group practice manager compensation rates are relatively low, exacerbating the challenge of hiring those with both experience and formal education.

Let's be clear: One does not need an MBA to successfully manage a small medical practice. In fact, a business degree may impede the achievement of someone with no experience. In best practice settings, however, great experience is accompanied by knowledge of business principles. Network executives need to build teams of practice managers who combine their daily operations expertise with a clear understanding of planning, organizing, staffing, directing, and controlling in a medical practice setting. Practice managers in hospital-owned settings need to be adept at managing physician sponsorship, organizing work, delegating responsibility, coaching, measuring performance, and holding teams and individuals accountable.

Medical practice managers need to become comfortable managing to a bottom line. They cannot be "storytellers," coming up with better excuses each month for budget variances. They need to be able to engage physicians and staff in developing and implementing tactics to drive performance improvement and achieve performance objectives. In our experience, managers with a high school diploma can be very successful in a hospital-owned practice with some additional supervisory training to learn the key principles of successful management. This combination of correct principles and real-world experience yields consistent performance.

Each location should be assigned a practice manager. Busy practices with several physicians/providers (three or more) and many employees (twelve or more) usually need a full-time manager just to oversee operations in this complex environment. Smaller practices can be clustered in two or three locations (depending on geographic proximity) and assigned to a shared or "cluster" manager. The cluster manager should be in each location each day for several hours and should be readily available by mobile phone when not present to manage. This approach allows even solo practices to benefit from the leadership of an experienced manager while sharing the costs with other practices.

Like other managers, practice managers need to have solid communication skills, be comfortable in a leadership role, and understand or be capable of understanding the principles of management and the basics of accounting and finance. A college degree is preferable, but it is not essential if the manager is willing to learn and the network executive is able to teach or arrange for education.

Director

As mentioned earlier, in best practice networks, network executives are physically in each practice frequently, preferably on a weekly basis, to observe and coach practice managers. Obviously, as networks grow and practice locations exceed ten, the network executive cannot physically spend adequate time in each location to effectively coach. Directors are operations experts (former seasoned practice managers are ideal) who report to the network executive and provide the oversight and coaching needed by practices and their managers.

Directors are assigned up to ten practice locations based on their ability to physically visit each location each week. They replace the network executive as members of the POCs in their assigned locations. Usually, organizations pursue directors with a master's degree in business, health care administration, or public administration and several years of hands-on experience.

Senior Executive

Some situations may arise in which the CEO–market manager is unable to consistently meet with his employed physician partners. In these cases the CEO may delegate authority for sponsoring the hospital-owned network to another senior hospital executive. Keys to successful delegation include the following:

1. Selecting an executive who has or will quickly gain a thorough understanding of the medical practice business
2. Delegating adequate authority to the senior executive to ensure that decisions made by the NOC, which includes the senior executive, cannot be undermined by an end-run to the CEO
3. Authorizing the senior executive to sign all physician employment agreements

Local System Structure

In markets where multiple affiliated hospitals form a local geographic system, managing their hospital-owned practices becomes complex. The structure and fundamental principles of the operational governance model remain the same, but because the market will have multiple CEO–market managers, and because market share strategy is primarily a local hospital function, management of the hospital-owned physician network must be sensitive to several levels of strategy.

For example, the local system will likely have some marketwide competitive strategies to meet community need and to position itself relative to competitors. Each hospital in the system will have certain strategies to ensure its long-term viability and competitive advantage by attracting adequate business from its primary service area. Both system and hospital strategies will be dependent, to a greater or lesser degree, on the employed physician network to capture market share in primary care practices and to refer that market share to affiliated specialists and hospitals when indicated.

The selection of many of the network's primary care and specialty physician strategies will likely be a function of those market share and service line objectives that originate at the system and hospitals. The employed network becomes the implementation arm for the local system. Consequently, hospital market managers in local systems are the "customers" of the network executive, who implements those portions of hospital strategy assigned to the employed physician network. The market managers accumulate capital, which is then usually distributed among the hospitals and the employed physician network by the local system CEO or senior market manager.

Staff Specialists

Managing the complexities of business is difficult without the assistance of specialists who have in-depth knowledge in a variety of fields. Human resource management, finance and accounting, risk and compliance, billing and coding, marketing, and health care law have become increasingly complex in recent years. Smaller organizations often depend on consultants in these disciplines, or go without that expertise.

Hospital-owned networks frequently have access to internal or contracted experts in these areas. This situation results in the the proverbial good news, bad news scenario. The good news is that these specialists can provide support to managers who are already consumed with the challenges of daily operations. Staff specialists recommend and establish policies to keep the organization, managers, and employees safe and compliant with law. They can provide relevant counsel based on in-depth knowledge of their areas of expertise; they can help managers become better managers.

The bad news involves four common problems with staff specialists:

1. *Role confusion.* Some staff specialists act like line managers. They forget that their role is to *support* line managers, who are (or should be) authorized to implement policies and procedures. They mistakenly believe their specialized knowledge, or external laws and regulations, authorize them to act. Some senior executives allow this behavior, the net affect of which is "the tail wagging the dog": Regulators, rather than physicians and managers, end up running the practice.
2. *The hammer.* "When your only tool is a hammer, everything looks like a nail." In-depth knowledge in any area creates a lens that biases the way experts see the world around them. That bias is essential in the proper context, but it often prevents a full understanding of circumstances necessary to make sound decisions.

3. *Relevance*. Similar to hospital administrators and managers, hospital staff experts may not understand the unique medical practice business. That lack of understanding makes it difficult for staff experts to apply their knowledge in this new setting. Some policies imposed on hospital-owned practices are irrelevant or, worse, hamper clinical quality, service quality, provider productivity, and financial viability.
4. *Accountability*. The ability to impose new policies, procedures, or change on a department or an organization should always be accompanied by accountability for the results of those decisions. Otherwise, the policy, procedure, or change is implemented in a vacuum, which can actually hamper outcomes and undermine line managers.

Staff specialists are essential in today's complex medical practice management world. These experts can maximize their contribution by remembering their role to support line managers and by taking time to learn the unique medical practice business as it relates to their area of expertise. They should always recommend policies and procedures based on that expertise, which are approved by the NOC and implemented by those who have line authority at the network and practice levels.

Summary

Critical success factors for the management infrastructure of a hospital-owned network include the following:

1. Viewing the management team, starting with the network executive, as implementers who take direction from the NOC for network-wide initiatives and from POCs for site-specific initiatives
2. Recognizing the role of the councils to hold physicians accountable rather than expecting managers to supervise employed physicians
3. Understanding the critical role of the hospital CEO as a market manager responsible for the success of each component of an integrated system, including primary care practices, specialty practices, ancillary services, hospital services, and hospital-based physicians
4. Selecting the right network executive and practice managers, ensuring that they have the knowledge, skills, and experience to implement initiatives at the network and site levels
5. Making sure that staff specialists understand their role as support for the NOC, the POCs, and the line managers rather than as managing the employed physician network

Close attention to these factors will ensure that the management infrastructure can function effectively for both the hospital and the physician network.

References

1. M. Halley, *The Primary Care–Market Share Connection: How Hospitals Achieve Competitive Advantage,* 11–12 (Chicago: Health Administration Press, 2007).

2. Ibid., 81–85.

3. Theodore Levitt, *The Marketing Imagination,* 119 (New York: Free Press, 1983).

4. Marc D. Halley and Robin L. Lloyd, "How to Break Even on an Acquired Primary Care Network," *Healthcare Financial Management* 54, no. 11 (2000): 69–74.

5. M. Halley and M. Ferry, *The Medical Practice Start-Up Guide* (Phoenix, MD: Greenbranch, 2008).

6. Kerry Patterson, Joseph Grenny, Ron McMillan, and Al Switzler, *Crucial Conversations: Tools for Talking When the Stakes Are High,* 3 (New York: McGraw-Hill, 2002).

CHAPTER 5

Network Development

We have discussed the role of the chief executive officer (CEO)–market manager as the logical strategic integrator. She is in the best position to partner with PCPs in capturing market share so that affiliated specialists and the hospital can attract that market share when clinically appropriate. The market manager also controls the capital-generating engine—the hospital—and determines how capital should be reinvested both within and outside the hospital walls to ensure the long-term viability of the integrated system.

As mentioned in chapter 1, many hospital executives are making the same mistakes now as were seen during phase 1 of physician employment. How, then, is a physician network developed properly to avoid these mistakes? Answering that question is the topic of this chapter.

Hospital performance dashboards frequently measure market share in terms of throughput. Admissions or cases are the result of referrals that come to the hospital primarily from primary care physicians (PCPs), specialists, and the hospital's emergency department. This hospital-centric measure of market share, however, is vulnerable to changes in those referral patterns. Primary care physicians may be hired by competing facilities. The hospital's top-producing surgeon might retire. Specialty physicians might open their own ambulatory surgery or diagnostic centers. Existing referral relationships might be circumvented by new PCPs or specialists entering the market. The hospital's own ancillary departments might become too busy to be accessible, driving business away.

Peter Drucker says the reason a business exists is to *create* and *keep* a customer.[1] Primary care physicians and internal medicine subspecialists treating chronic disease keep customers in the form of active patients. "My doctor" for most of the population refers to a PCP. Successful specialists and hospitals are dependent on their relationships with these referring providers. Specialty physicians (particularly invasive specialists) and hospitals are "occurrence" providers because the service they provide typically spans a short time frame.[2] The only way for hospitals and many specialists to create and keep a customer is to maintain referral relationships.

Network development includes the following key components, each of which requires the time and personal attention of the market manager:

- A solid primary care "retail" strategy based on clear geographic and market share targets

- An effective strategy for connecting primary care physicians with affiliated specialists
- An effective strategy for connecting both PCPs and specialists with the hospital and its services (demand chain management)
- An effective and efficient physician recruitment process
- An effective and efficient practice acquisition process

In the past, many hospitals have employed physicians either as a *reaction* to competitive moves or to requests from established physicians or as a physician recruitment tool. Today, increasing numbers of hospitals and health systems are employing physicians as a *proactive* competitive strategy, with a focus on capturing market share or attracting referrals from those who hold market share.

Capturing or retaining market share is largely dictated by primary care physicians and the long-term relationships they develop with their patients. We define retail strategy as placing PCPs conveniently throughout a hospital's service area. Attracting referrals from primary care and other referring physicians in competitive settings includes becoming the specialist of choice[3] and the hospital of choice. Hospitals have commonly used a service line strategy to attract specialists and patient referrals to the hospital workshop. Today's competitive markets require those same specialists and hospital service lines to cooperate and become demand chains, working as a unit to build and retain referral relationships.

Retail Strategy

During the discussion of retail strategy and demand chain management we make reference to the book *The Primary Care–Market Share Connection: How Hospitals Achieve Competitive Advantage*, published by Health Administration Press in 2007.[4] It proposes that, in the absence of a preexisting condition, when "Mrs. Smith" (who makes the majority of health care decisions for the family) moves to town, she chooses to obtain medical services for her family from among the four key "relationship" primary care medical specialties: family medicine, general internal medicine, pediatrics, and obstetrics. She will most likely select that PCP based on a recommendation from a neighbor, friend, or relative, who will likely recommend her own physician. If Mrs. Smith lives in an urban or suburban area, she prefers to find the family's doctor within a short drive of home and schools for convenience, especially if she works outside the home.

Mrs. Smith tends to build a long-term relationship with her selected primary care physician(s). Importantly, she is usually dependent on that trusted PCP to recommend a specialist in the event that specialty service is needed. Her PCP can also have significant influence over her selection of a hospital, either directly, through referring or admitting the patient for ancillary or inpatient services, or indirectly, through referring to an affiliated specialty physician for an inpatient or outpatient procedure.

While Mrs. Smith prefers her PCP to be close to home, she will often drive further—even across town and against natural migration patterns—to see a specialist referred by her PCP. Based on our experience helping clients attract/redirect referrals, this phenomenon appears to be a function of several factors:

- *Perceived value*. A referral to a specialty physician often means that "I am really sick." Consequently, the "utility" or perceived value of the specialty visit is high—at least initially.
- *Decision information*. It is unlikely that I came to my primary care visit having researched options for the specialty my PCP will recommend. My PCP will likely refer me to the specialist of his choice, based on his past referral experience with that specialist. His preference will likely be based on factors such as access to the specialist, communication with the specialist, and feedback from previously referred patients.
- *Trust*. Patients tend to trust the judgment of their PCP in selecting the best specialist for their illness, condition, injury, or circumstance. Unless the patient is personally acquainted with a specialty physician alternative (e.g., "Dr. Case replaced my mother's hip"), the PCP's recommendation will likely be accepted.
- *Mobility*. If I am mobile (I own a reliable vehicle) and family members who may need to accompany me are mobile, I am more able and willing to follow my PCP's advice to see a specialist across town rather than asking for a different specialist located closer to my home.

Understanding these basic principles and validating them in the local market are critical steps for the successful market manager as he considers developing a retail strategy.

All practices that provide primary care services can be considered retail practices because they serve the ultimate user—the patient. She can self-select primary care medical services like other retail services and develops shopping or loyalty patterns based largely on her satisfaction with the convenience, access, and service quality she experiences. Like most people, Mrs. Smith assumes that she will find clinical quality at these locations, and clinical quality only becomes an issue in her decision to select or return to a practice when it is obviously absent. This concept is more fully explored in chapter 6.

A market manager who understands retail strategy will want to ensure that his hospital has adequate numbers of employed or affiliated PCPs in all the suitable neighborhoods in the primary and secondary target markets for the hospital or integrated delivery system. For our purposes, a primary care neighborhood includes all the households within about a ten-minute drive (about a five-mile radius) of an urban or suburban primary care medical practice location. These households usually account for between 50 and 75 percent of active patients in the primary care practice. (Women living in rural areas will routinely drive much further than ten minutes away for retail services, including a PCP visit.) A viable primary care practice may capture between 2,000 and 5,000 active patients per physician.

What are the right neighborhoods? A retail analysis will help the market manager determine the answer to that question.

Based on Mrs. Smith's preferences for the family's physician, geographic placement of PCPs is very important, especially in competitive markets. Being "first" in a neighborhood is also important given the family's health care decision maker's tendency to stay with her selected PCP. Wise market managers understand that the geographic placement of employed and affiliated PCPs in urban and suburban settings will affect the demographic, psychographic, household income, and payer profiles of patients seen by affiliated specialists and those patients admitted to the hospital. For example, newer neighborhoods of starter homes tend to attract young families. Neighborhoods with custom homes tend to attract households that are more established, many with two income producers. Some neighborhoods attract only well-established households with significant income levels. Others attract those that are likely to struggle to make ends meet.

Market managers can target these various neighborhoods by first locating family physicians within easy access. As market share is captured in these practices, market managers can add other providers to meet the needs of that market, including internists, pediatricians, and obstetricians (although women tell us they will drive further for the right obstetrician/gynecologist). Larger diagnostic centers and specialty practices can be conveniently located to support a number of neighborhoods and PCPs on, for example, the "east side" or "west side."

Launching a retail strategy includes the following steps:

- Developing a clear primary and secondary market definition based not only on current admissions but also on desired market share and geographies served, and comparing that target with the current throughput (admissions) by zip code
- Understanding the underlying population demographic and psychographic trends affecting the primary and secondary markets
- Identifying the primary care practices in the area, as well as their affiliation, which will help answer the following critical questions:
  —Where are the organization's current and potential market share?
  —Who is holding it (by physician name)?
  —What are they doing with it?
- Identifying the development of retail corridors in the market (watch the growth of retailers like Walgreens, CVS/pharmacy, and other entities that use specific geographic strategies to effectively saturate markets)

- Identifying statistical community need for various PCP specialties
- Combining all the above data to yield the following growth targets by zip code:
  —Neighborhoods where additional primary care capacity is needed or where existing physician capacity is nearing retirement and will need to be replaced
  —Neighborhoods where markets are saturated but PCPs are working for or affiliated with the competitor
  —Neighborhoods where the population is growing or projected to grow rapidly
  —Neighborhoods where the population would improve the hospital's payer mix
  —Neighborhoods where the population is underserved
- Developing tactics, including the following:
  —The addition of new physician capacity to specific zip codes to maintain (replacement tactics) or capture additional market share
  —The acquisition of targeted practices to protect market share
  —The acquisition of targeted practices to increase market share
  —The development of mission-based practices to improve access to the underserved
- Prioritizing tactics and implementation based on available capital

Most of the information necessary to complete a retail analysis is readily available or can be purchased for a relatively small fee. The process of analysis is straightforward; market managers need not guess about the best locations to start or acquire primary care facilities.

Becoming the Specialist of Choice

Specialists of choice are those specialty physicians who understand that referring physicians are their most important customer—even more important than the patients they refer. Why? It is unlikely that Mrs. Smith self-selected the specialist and even less likely that she will diagnose and refer anyone else. Certainly, failure to treat Mrs. Smith properly will result in negative feedback to the referring physician, which is the death knell for future referrals. But because the referring physician is trained to diagnose and refer Mrs. Smith and her neighbors, he or she is the specialist's most important customer.

Wise specialty physicians understand that patient referrals are subject to two basic tenets:[5]

- Referrals follow relationships.
- All relationships atrophy over time.

Referring physicians repeatedly tell us what factors motivate them to refer patients to a particular specialist; they include the following:

- *Access.* I can ensure that the patient (particularly an anxious patient) is seen by the specialty physician in a timely manner.
- *Communication.* I am able to communicate with the specialist on my terms. I may want to talk with the specialist in advance of the visit or consultation, or I may only want an update after the visit.
- *Relationship management.* The specialist engages me in the treatment planning process and is willing to share his or her specific expertise with me as a professional. The specialist returns the patient to me.
- *Previous referral experience.* My patients are pleased with the way they were treated by the specialist and his or her support staff.

Interestingly, we do not often see the specialist's *clinical competence* at the top of the list of motivators. When we ask referring physicians why, they tell us that clinical competence is assumed. It only becomes an issue when it is not present. In addition, clinical competence is often difficult to measure. It would be a challenge for most referring physicians to pick the most technically competent cardiologist or general surgeon in their community. Otherwise, one specialist would have all the business and the rest would starve. Referrals do, then, follow relationships.

Why do these important referral relationships atrophy over time? Consider the following common scenario. Dr. Jones, a brand new neurologist, comes to town, joins the medical staff of a local hospital, and opens an office on campus. The hospital announces his arrival with the traditional newspaper advertisements and facilitates his introduction to potential referring physicians. Within a few days he receives his first referral from Dr. Case. Dr. Jones is readily available to schedule the patient (one of only four patients scheduled that day) and to immediately take Dr. Case's call regarding the referring physician's objectives for the consultation. Dr. Jones sees the patient immediately and spends plenty of time diagnosing, treating, and educating her. He then creates a clear and concise written summary of the visit, which is forwarded to Dr. Case electronically within twenty-four hours of the visit. Dr. Jones follows up with Dr. Case and the patient by telephone shortly after the visit to make sure that the expectations of each have been met.

Dr. Jones' reputation as an accessible, affable, and capable clinician spreads quickly. Soon his practice is booming. He now sees twenty, thirty, or more patients per day and experiences a three-week wait for a new patient consult. He has a difficult time returning all of his referring physicians' telephone calls the same day and rarely contacts a patient after a visit. His consultation documentation is clinically adequate but noticeably brief. Dr. Case is now one of twenty-five physicians who regularly refer patients to Dr. Jones—many of whom the specialist has not met face-to-face because they never come to the hospital, which has a

24/7 hospitalist program. He is no longer accessible and is too busy to be affable, even though his clinical skills are adequate. He still loves what he is doing, but he is weary—and so are his staff members.

Dr. Jones' referring physicians have now become vulnerable to an astute competitor, who is, or appears to be, more accessible, more affable, and so forth. This scenario is common for successful practices, but it can be managed to reduce the vulnerability of losing referring physicians. As they become busier, smart specialists understand that paying attention to the details of practice operations is critical to success in maintaining relationships with referral sources. Their support staff, technology capabilities, job design, customer service training and scripting, policies and procedures, processes, productivity, and more can help them maintain their relationships with referring physicians. We discuss these concepts more fully in subsequent chapters.

Demand Chain Strategy

In the past, many service lines followed the same "build it and they will come" approach as other hospital departments. The organization built new space, bought new equipment, hired a medical director, wooed existing specialists, and recruited new ones, hoping to fill the operating rooms and beds. More recently, many hospitals have employed the specialists in hopes of locking in the business, only to discover, once again, that specialists, particularly invasive specialists, do not control market share.

Certainly, the service line model has successfully differentiated some hospitals from competitors, particularly in certificate-of-need states that limit redundancy. The service line model has clearly yielded clinical quality and process improvements in many cases. From a market share perspective, however, being one of five heart programs, or three cancer centers, or four orthopedic hospitals in a market is hardly a recipe for distinction—with or without billboards announcing their existence. Some hospitals have discovered that their service lines and new employed specialists are under-differentiated and underutilized.

A demand chain is more than a service line.[6] It is a partnership linking the hospital-based specialists with relevant hospital departments, specialty physicians, and PCPs. A demand chain is built around meeting the needs, wants, and priorities of referring physicians and their patients. In fact, an effective demand chain is built on those factors that "wow" referring physicians and their patients.* For example, a heart hospital and its employed specialty physicians (one of several community heart programs) decided to differentiate themselves in terms of

*I am indebted to Joann Anderson and her team at Southeastern Regional Medical Center, who use the term *wow* to describe their commitment to the customer. This simple term is the essence of an effective demand chain.

service. The specialists and hospital administration surveyed PCPs to understand what factors motivated referrals to the specialists and the hospital. The specialists and administration then met with representative PCPs face-to-face and discussed survey results. Based on the information gathered, the cardiologists realized that access was a key motivator for PCPs to refer. They learned that when a PCP uses the "C" word ("cardiologist") with a patient, the patient's anxiety level and blood pressure immediately rise. Part of that anxiety is an urgency to be seen immediately by the specialist.

In response, the cardiologists developed a plan to offer open-access scheduling every weekday afternoon to help ensure same-day service for referring physicians and their patients. They also committed to a system whereby the cardiologist on call would personally see a patient after hours at the request of the referring physician—even if the problem did not appear to be urgent. The cardiology group worked with the hospital staff to develop a process for turning around test results within twenty-four hours rather than forty-eight hours. Small gestures like these "wow" referring physicians.

Bringing hospital-based physicians, hospital departments, specialists, and PCPs together to focus on identifying and meeting the needs, wants, and priorities of referring physicians and their patients is the essence of demand chain management. Ensuring that organizations wow PCPs, referring specialists, and their patients takes cooperation among physicians and hospital departments, all of which are focused on the customer. Further, it takes a service commitment—a promise that goes beyond clinical quality, as quality is usually assumed for every heart program, cancer center, and other specialty practice.

Market Management

Astute market managers understand that they must attract and retain enough PCPs to capture the market share they need to support their affiliated specialists and the capital-generating hospital. More so now than in the past, whether these physicians are employed or are independent and brand-loyal matters, especially when hospital executives in highly competitive markets realize that independent, even brand-loyal, PCPs are vulnerable to hostile takeover. In addition, long-standing referral patterns for hospital-employed PCPs are increasingly modified by "domestic" referral mandates issued by competing market managers in order to support their increasing numbers of hospital-employed specialists.

More and more hospital executives understand that PCPs capture, hold, and direct their market share. They recognize that employing a significant number of them is the best way to build a sustainable competitive advantage. They also recognize that engaging specialists of choice and hospital departments as effective demand chains is the best way to attract patient referrals from employed or independent physicians.

Most market managers find it necessary to develop an employment model just to recruit new physicians to the medical staff. Many are finding it necessary to develop an employed physician network to remain competitive in the marketplace. Some hospital CEOs have focused on employing specialists and strengthening their service lines. This one-dimensional model, however, can always be trumped by a competitor focused on capturing, retaining, and directing market share through employed PCPs.

In the midst of these competitive realities, some market managers wonder how to balance physician employment and competitive pressures with the need to maintain relationships with independent physicians, both PCPs and specialists. We encourage our hospital clients to develop and maintain productive relationships with as many physicians as possible, regardless of their current employment status. Hospitals should be prepared to successfully engage physicians in multiple ways, depending on the preference of these valuable customers.

Figure 5-1 illustrates the five common physician integration approaches, each of which should be a successful part of a hospital's repertoire. Independent physicians who simply want a workshop should be welcomed to the medical staff and hospital of choice. Those interested in building a program with the organization may be engaged as medical directors or members of the service line teams and demand chains (to be discussed later). Some physicians are interested in joint venturing with the hospital. (Effective joint ventures do not simply shift hospital revenue to physicians. Instead, they increase the size of the market share pie in order to protect both parties.) Some physicians want to maintain their independence but are willing to contract with the hospital to provide services. Finally, an increasing number of physicians want a hospital employment option.

Figure 5-1. Common Integration Options

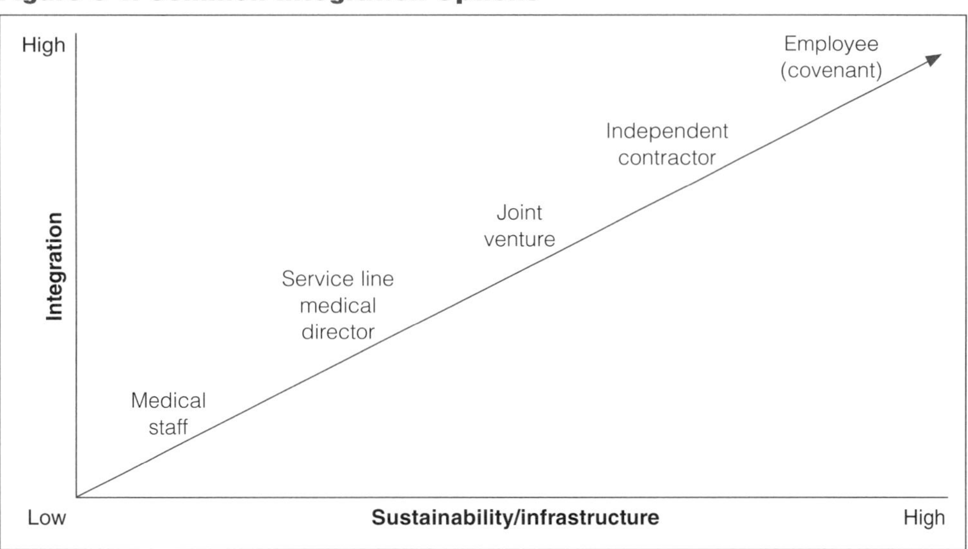

Wise market managers ensure that their hospital can successfully implement all five approaches, recognizing that physicians may move up or down the integration scale over time. Employed physicians are encouraged to refer to and share call with independent physicians who are affiliated or willing to be affiliated with the organization. We encourage employed physicians to refer to both independent and employed specialists, but to make it clear that procedures should be performed in their capital-generating hospital(s).

Potential Impact of Employed and Affiliated Physicians

The financial value of physician utilization of hospital services has been the subject of debate for years. A recent survey conducted by Merritt Hawkins asked hospital chief financial officers to provide the average inpatient and outpatient net revenue for several specialties derived through their direct referrals. Annual net revenue for three specialties was reported as follows:

- Internal medicine: $1,987,253
- Family medicine: $1,615,828
- Pediatrics: $697,516

These figures include values provided for direct primary care referrals only. No indirect referrals to specialists were included. The value of other specialty physician net revenue ranged from a high of $2,662,600 for invasive cardiologists to a low of $557,916 for neurologists. The average for all specialty physicians (including obstetrics/gynecology) was $1,509,910 in 2007.[7]

While hospitals cannot legally pay physicians for referrals or downstream revenues, the value of physician referrals and utilization of the hospital is clear. Also clear from the 2007 survey is that value is decreasing since the last Merritt Hawkins survey in 2004, when the average specialty net revenue was $1,885,773.[8] This phenomenon may be a function of changes in technology facilitating new office-based services, changing reimbursement, competing physician-owned diagnostic and ambulatory surgery facilities, or other factors. Regardless of the reasons for the decrease in value, the trend illustrates the importance of understanding and managing *where* market share is captured or retained and *how* it migrates through the health care system generating both revenue and capital.

It is also important to realize that $1.5 million in annual net patient revenue per physician translates to about $45,000 in operating capital, assuming a 3 percent bottom line. The combined efforts of employed and independent medical staff members can generate significant capital. At the same time, a hospital-owned medical practice network losing millions annually can consume a substantial portion of that capital, which might be put to better strategic use.

Growth Tactics

A primary care retail analysis is usually a subset of a strategic medical staff development plan. Retail analysis goes beyond simply identifying community need, to determining competitive tactics. For example, in a zip code already saturated with PCPs, the hospital must target and acquire existing practices rather than add more capacity. In an area teeming with excess demand for services, such as a rapidly growing neighborhood or an underserved community, the hospital may elect to cold start a new practice.

In a zip code where additional capacity is needed but brand-loyal physicians are already present, starting a new, competing practice may not be perceived favorably by the established group. Instead, the hospital could consider initiating a "side by side" arrangement, which places employed physicians alongside established physicians in practice for the benefit of all parties. In this contractual arrangement, the new employed physicians expand capacity in the zip code as part of the established group and provide additional on-call coverage. The hospital absorbs a share of the practice's fixed and variable overhead. The practice is obligated to treat the new physicians as partners in terms of sharing new patients, providing adequate support staffing, sharing billing services, and so forth. The hospital usually asks for a right of first refusal should the independent group decide to sell the practice.

Regardless of the tactics used (and most hospitals will use all of them at one time or another), the hospital will likely need to define and potentially implement two very important processes: physician recruitment and practice acquisition.

Successful Physician Recruitment Is Key to Retention

Experienced physician recruiters know that many new physicians are not very sophisticated in selecting their first practice opportunity when leaving a residency or fellowship training program. In fact, a great time to "steal" young physicians is eighteen to twenty-four months after they start their first job.

An article published by Merritt Hawkins entitled "Summary Report: 2005 Survey of Hospital Physician Recruitment Trends" cites a study conducted by the Department of Health Science at Towson University.[9] It examined turnover rates among younger PCPs, looking at employed PCPs younger than forty-five who had been in practice between two and nine years. The study showed that over a five-year period, 55 percent of these physicians had left the practice in which they were originally employed. Twenty percent of physicians in the study group had left two employers in five years.

Forty-six percent of physicians who leave their practices are most likely to do so within the first three years, according to a 2008 Cejka Search/American

Medical Group Association survey.[10] The same survey found that those physicians who voluntarily resigned from a practice identified the following reason(s) (*Cejka Search/AMGA 2008 Physician Retention Survey*. © 2009, American Medical Group Association. www.amga.org):

- 50 percent cited a poor cultural fit
- 32 percent relocated to be closer to family
- 26 percent were seeking higher compensation
- 22 percent were pursuing a better community fit
- 18 percent cited a spouse job relocation
- 8 percent identified an incompatible work schedule
- 6 percent indicated excessive call requirements

In the face of these realities, physician recruitment can only be considered successful if the "right" physician is recruited and retained. Selecting the "wrong" candidate or one who leaves within months can cost the employing health care network far more than the recruiting fee. Consider the original sunk costs associated with the departing physician's recruitment and practice start-up. Consider also the lost patient base and downstream revenues, as at least a portion of the practice's patients will usually leave when their doctor leaves. Finally, consider new recruiting costs and the replacement physician's start-up expenses, which can easily exceed $200,000 for a PCP during the first year.

Effective and efficient physician recruitment includes several key steps:

1. Candidate sourcing
2. Opportunity development
3. Candidate assessment
4. Negotiation
5. Operational start-up

Many hospitals pay little attention to steps 1 and 5 and simply stumble through steps 2, 3, and 4. Others assume that if they hire a professional physician recruitment firm, they need not worry about the process at all. But success, particularly in competitive specialties, requires careful attention to each step whether an internal or external recruitment professional is engaged. Each step is discussed below.

Candidate Sourcing

For those hospitals with only occasional recruitment needs, candidate sourcing usually includes a contract with an outside recruitment firm that is constantly sourcing physician candidates in a variety of specialties. For those hospitals (and increasingly for those health systems) that have multiple and continuous recruitment needs over several years, candidate sourcing usually justifies an internal recruiting resource. That internal resource will typically handle most candidate sourcing, although he or she may still use outside recruiters to source difficult-to-find specialists.

Many hospitals have found that physician retention is heavily influenced by local geographic ties. Physicians who have family, training, or other connections in or near a particular geographic area are more likely to remain in that market for the long term, sometimes even forgoing potentially higher incomes elsewhere. For this reason, building relationships with local and regional residency programs is a high priority for hospitals. Residency program relationship tactics include the following:

- Hosting a residency program on campus, which may provide a huge competitive advantage for a hospital or health system by building geographic ties, hospital ties, and ties with specialists and by giving the recruiter "first shot" at the best candidates each year.
- Building relationships with the residency directors, who can guide recruiters to the top candidates each year.
- Hosting annual dinners, with a "selecting your medical practice" theme, for residents (including first-year) and their spouses or significant others to position the recruiter and the hospital as the experts in the selection process.
- Providing practice start-up and management training sessions, including management professionals and practicing physicians among the instructors. Even those physicians seeking an employment option need to understand that the day they leave their residency program they are *in business*—even as employees. We often hear residents say "I just want to practice medicine" (leaving the business decisions to someone else). We remind them that if they do not understand and cannot contribute to business decisions affecting their selected practice, someone else will make those decisions, which will affect their clinical practice and quality of work life.[†]
- Becoming a sounding board by offering to help residents talk through their practice opportunities, even for those who are clearly leaving the area. They will refer their peers and underclassmates to you, some of whom will want to remain local.
- Attending or helping to sponsor local and regional recruitment fairs.
- Working with state medical associations to sponsor practice management or practice selection sessions.

---

†Our medical practice start-up guide was created for this very purpose. See M. Halley and M. Ferry, eds., *The Medical Practice Start-Up Guide* (Phoenix, MD: Greenbranch, 2008).

In addition to residency relationships, internal recruiters can look to recently recruited physicians for referrals of underclassmates. Trusting relationships are often built among residents during training programs. An invitation from a trusted friend who has had a great experience with your hospital and your medical group or medical staff is a superb sourcing technique.

The Internet continues to emerge as a significant source for physician candidates, most of whom are part of the "Facebook generation" for whom social networking is a normal part of life. A number of recruitment Web sites and Internet advertising options may be considered. Several Internet-based organizations allow, for a fee, various levels of "matching" for physician candidates and those organizations with job opportunities. Of course, the traditional method of posting opportunities in publications is still available, as well.

Regardless of the methods selected (and most hospitals will use several), sourcing the right candidates starts with the right type of sourcing activities. The most successful of those activities involve opportunities to build relationships with candidates even before they are considering job options.

Opportunity Development

Another very important part of the physician recruitment process, and one that is critical to selecting the right candidate, is opportunity development. Opportunity development starts with a thorough analysis of the market potential for the new physician (e.g., retail analysis, strategic medical staff development planning). It also includes cultivation of the practice opportunity. For example, would an established group practice consider accommodating the new candidate or at least sharing call coverage with her? Where will the new office be located? What is the hospital willing to offer in terms of pay and benefits or an income guarantee (which is no longer very effective, even with loan forgiveness)? Will a signing bonus be offered? Who will manage the start-up process with the new physician, including credentialing (medical staff and payers) and the new practice start-up action plan? In short, what specifically is "the deal" the recruiter is authorized to offer?

Once these and myriad other questions have been answered, the practice opportunity can be documented in a practice opportunity prospectus. The prospectus is a sales document that clearly articulates the opportunity and keeps those involved in the interview process on the same track when they discuss that opportunity with potential candidates. A prospectus is approved in advance by the hospital CEO, so no surprises arise for interested candidates or recruiters.

While a practice opportunity prospectus for an established practice would be different from that of a cold-start opportunity, in general, it may contain several of the following elements:

- *Practice vision.* The vision of the established physicians, if joining a group, or the vision of hospital administration, if starting a new practice, should be clearly documented. Obviously, the more compelling the vision, the easier it is to sell the opportunity to the right candidate. A compelling practice vision is an essential part of finding and retaining the right new physician.

- *Practice history.* If applicable, a brief history of an established practice gives potential candidates perspective about existing physicians and the development of the practice. Longevity, stability, innovation, and other historical factors should be important considerations for new physicians looking to join an established group.
- *Physician biographies.* If applicable, biographical statements about the established physicians in a practice will be of interest to potential candidates.
- *Staff biographies.* If applicable, biographical statements about the support staff in an established practice will be of interest to serious potential candidates.
- *Location and facilities.* Identifying the benefits of the practice location and a description of existing or proposed facilities is tangible evidence that the hospital is serious about the opportunity. Ideally, show the candidate her personal office space and start discussing office furniture allowances and her preferences.
- *Area demographics.* Discussing openly why the organization needs to add physician capacity in this particular specialty is a critical part of the prospectus. Is the need based on significant community demand, or will the hospital be battling for market share with competing specialists? The practice pro forma will reflect these market realities.
- *Practice performance.* Always include key financial and statistical benchmarks for the candidate to review. If a physician candidate is not interested in discussing practice financial and statistical performance, she is probably not the ideal partner. The fact that you do discuss those realities is much appreciated by most candidates, who realize that they will be expected to participate in ensuring the success of the enterprise—even as employees.
- *Practice opportunity.* Clearly spelling out the compensation and benefits is essential. Detailing it in advance sets the candidate's expectations and keeps the organization grounded during the interview and negotiation process. A critical component of the practice opportunity is a high-level pro forma estimating how the practice will develop, identifying the investment that will be required, and establishing a realistic timeline to financial viability.
- *Associated hospital and health system.* Presenting the affiliated hospital(s) and the health system, if appropriate, can be an important part of convincing the candidate that it is the right hospital partner.

- *Community*. Many recruitment decisions include factors beyond the practice itself. Preferred neighborhoods, recreational activities, spousal job opportunities, schools, cultural events, and many other factors influence the decision to choose an opportunity and to "stay and play" for the long term.

The practice opportunity prospectus is usually fifteen to twenty pages in length and is presented with a professional cover sheet and low-profile spiral binding.

The planning process forces the hospital to get its recruitment act together and serves as a reminder to the candidate of the opportunity long after the magic of the site visit has faded. Still, many organizations do not take the time to prepare this short document—a simple yet powerful way to distinguish your offer.

Candidate Assessment

Assessing candidates is critical to recruiting and retaining the right individual. As mentioned earlier, the loss involved in a recruiting mistake can be hundreds of thousands of dollars in recruitment costs, initial practice operating losses, and the loss of market share as patients (or referring physicians) scramble for a replacement physician. Special attention should be paid to the assessment of each candidate and should include the following steps:

1. Initial contact
2. Telephone interview
3. Site visit
4. Reference check
5. Relationship development

INITIAL CONTACT

The purpose of the initial contact is to allow both parties to determine if the potential exists for a match between the candidate's key objectives and the practice opportunity. It is a high-level discussion and an opportunity to get acquainted and to start building relationships. The relationship between the candidate and the recruiter is critical and begins with this first contact, which is usually by telephone.

TELEPHONE INTERVIEW

If both parties remain interested after the first telephone contact, an in-depth telephone or face-to-face (for local candidates) interview is scheduled. During the interview, the recruiter shares additional details about the practice opportunity, usually without discussing the terms of the deal.

We recommend using a specifically developed candidate interview form that includes a series of questions relating to the candidate's objectives, training, and experience. The candidate interview form we use is found in Appendix C. (Although this form has been reviewed by human resource professionals, we encourage recruiters to make sure it does not violate any legal or regulatory issues as interpreted by your human resources department and legal counsel.) The interview form provides a consistent platform for gathering information to assess the potential for a match between possible candidates and a practice opportunity.

SITE VISIT

If the candidate and the recruiter feel the opportunity exists for a match, a site visit is scheduled. It may include family members who have their own objectives for the visit. Helping the spouse and children address these issues is critical to the recruitment and retention process.

The site visit should ideally include interviews with physicians of the same specialty, physicians practicing in the same or similar circumstances, referring physicians (if applicable), administrative leaders, and those who will be responsible for successfully on-boarding the new physician. We recommend that the recruiter attend all these interviews to hear what questions are asked and responses made, ensuring that questions and answers are appropriate and legal. Ideally, feedback from interviewees should be pursued immediately after the visit via telephone call, e-mail, or formal score sheet. The site visit may also include time with a real estate agent and other community representatives who can authoritatively respond to relevant questions the physician, spouse, and children may have.

The practice opportunity prospectus is provided to the candidate during the interview with the signatory or during the exit interview with the recruiter. The exit interview is an important step to ensure that questions and objectives have been addressed and next steps clarified. Depending on the situation, a formal offer letter and term sheet may be prepared and provided during the exit interview, or this step may be delayed if feedback from interviewers is not yet collected.

REFERENCE CHECK

All offers and discussions should be made contingent on successful reference checking by the medical staff office. In addition to ensuring references are checked for credentialing purposes, the recruiter should make sure that behavioral references are pursued.

RELATIONSHIP DEVELOPMENT

Assuming the parties are still interested after the site visit, the recruiter should ensure that consistent follow-up occurs. Once the candidate receives a formal offer, the negotiation process has commenced. That process may be protracted if the candidate is considering other locations and offers. Getting the candidate's permission to periodically "check in" helps build relationships and will provide insights into competitive offerings. The relationship development process includes selected physicians and administration, but the most important voice in the process is the recruiter.

Negotiation

Negotiation is the next component of the recruitment process. We have found that having a negotiator other than the hospital signatory is a best practice. Most often, that negotiator is the recruiter, who assumes the role of helping both parties successfully complete the transaction. Although the recruiter works for the hospital, if retention is clearly as important as recruitment, everyone has the incentive to do the *right deal* with the *right physician*. Such "arms length" negotiation allows the signatory parties space and time to thoughtfully negotiate by weighing those few terms and conditions that might be allowed to vary. For example, the signing bonus may be increased, the moving allowance may differ, or the start date may be modified.

We prefer to start the negotiation process with a formal offer letter and an attached term sheet that addresses the most often asked questions from candidates, as opposed to sending the candidate away with twenty or thirty pages of legalese. A sample term sheet is provided in Appendix D.

Once the highlights of the term sheet, including potentially "scary" items like a covenant not to compete, have been discussed, the contract can be reviewed during a one-on-one discussion between the trusted recruiter and the physician candidate.

Operational Start-Up

Finally, and importantly, retention is significantly influenced by an efficient and effective start-up process, which includes physician mentoring and numerous other start-up activities. The Halley Consulting Group's generic medical practice start-up action plan is provided in Appendix E.

The start-up process ideally begins six months in advance of the new physician's first day on the job. It can be completed in less time, but consequences are inherent in short-cutting the process (e.g., payer credentialing and delayed or lost reimbursement for services initially performed).

The implementation team that supports the start-up process includes those staff experts and line managers who will help ensure the success of the new physician and/or practice. The process is driven by line managers, and the team usually meets at least every other week, depending on the volume of work. Representatives from finance, human resources, billing/credentialing, information technology, marketing and communications, and other areas are likely participants.

Effective Practice Acquisition

As soon as the hospital employs that first physician or acquires that first practice, the CEO should be prepared to field inquiries from others interested in affiliation. The first to pursue an arrangement are likely to be those physicians who are unable to succeed on their own. Often, those are not the physicians a hospital wants to attract as business partners. If they cannot succeed in practice on their own, it is unlikely that they will be effective upon being employed by a hospital. Instead, market managers should proactively identify those practices with whom the hospital wants to do business because the physicians are also successful businessmen and -women. Those practices and physicians are likely to include both offensive (pursuing new market share) and defensive (protecting existing market share) targets.

Once target practices have been identified, the relationship development and management process begins in earnest. Even if the targeted physicians are not ready to join the hospital team, they should become part of the market manager's relationship management process, as discussed earlier in this chapter.

If a targeted physician or group expresses interest in selling the practice, the hospital should have an organized process in place for evaluation and decision making. That process should include the steps described below.

Practice Evaluation

A practice evaluation is a thorough examination of several areas of business administration and includes answering a number of questions, such as those that follow:

- *Operational governance.* Do the physicians have a demonstrated track record of making, and working with their manager to successfully implement, decisions? Do the physicians hold each other accountable to comply with group decisions?
- *Management effectiveness.* How competent is the practice manager? Does he or she have the respect of physicians and support staff? How would he or she fit in with the hospital's network management structure?
- *Practice marketing.* What are the image and reputation of the practice and the physicians? Is the practice a growing concern, with the right new patient ratio (for PCPs) or a solid corps of referring physicians (for specialty physicians)? What do patient satisfaction scores reveal?
- *Human resource issues.* Are staff members well trained? Are wages and benefits in line with those offered by the hospital-owned network? How will current physician productivity translate to the network physician compensation model?
- *Practice operations.* Are operations well organized? Is staffing appropriate, and is the team well trained? Is the practice applying highest and best-use staffing models? Is physician productivity a priority? How are clinical quality and service quality issues addressed in the practice?

- *Receivables management.* Are the accounts receivable in good shape? How strong are point-of-service collections? What does the coding index look like for each physician? What percentage of claims are clean? What are contractual write-offs as a percentage of charges?
- *Information technology.* How effective is the practice management software? Is the software the latest version? Are all modules functional? What is the age of the computer hardware? Does the practice have a full or partial electronic medical record system (EMR)? How efficient and effective is the EMR? Is the software up to date?
- *Physical facilities and equipment.* Is the facility clean and professional in appearance? Are furnishings functional and in good repair? Is equipment (clinical and business) functional and in good repair?
- *Financial and statistical performance.* How does practice performance compare with national benchmarks? Are the physicians conscious of their own performance and its contribution to practice performance? What are the trends in each revenue and expense category?

A practice evaluation yields a series of findings and recommendations, which are documented for use by both parties. Based on those findings, the parties may choose to continue discussions or not. If not, the physicians will still come away with a valuable set of recommendations in return for their willingness to participate in the process.

Practice Valuation

If both parties choose to continue pursuing a possible acquisition, the next step is to conduct a practice valuation. The valuation involves attaching a value to various components of the medical practice. We recommend selecting a qualified third party to conduct the valuation. That third party will benefit from and should receive a copy of the practice evaluation.

The valuator will likely examine real property, furnishings, and equipment associated with the practice. He may also value the accounts receivable at an appropriate discount. Other aspects of the practice may receive his attention, as well.

Most hospitals no longer pay for the value of a going concern (sometimes called goodwill). Some valuators use the Internal Revenue Service–approved discounted cash flow method to assign a value to the practice. Frequently, the valuation company will provide the value in terms of a range.

Negotiation

If the valuation range seems reasonable to the parties, the process can continue. As with the recruitment process, we recommend the use of a term sheet to present the key terms and conditions of the deal. In the case of acquisition, the deal may include multiple components, such as the acquisition of all or certain practice assets, engagement of the physicians as employees or as independent contractors, and a lease agreement for assets (usually real property) the physicians choose to retain. Contracts for each component must be developed by competent legal counsel.

In a well-functioning hospital-owned medical practice network, the network executive is in an excellent position to serve as the chief negotiator on behalf of the hospital CEO, who will ultimately sign the agreements. As the person who will ultimately be responsible for the successful operation and integration of the new practice, the network executive's early involvement reduces the potential for unsustainable promises and unfulfilled side conversations.

Transition Action Plan

As with employing new physicians, using a detailed action plan in the acquisition of a practice will reduce the number of blunders likely to occur during the transition process. An implementation team, working under the direction of the network executive, develops a transition action plan similar to the start-up action plan discussed earlier.

The implementation team includes staff experts from finance, human resources, billing/credentialing, information technology, and marketing and communications as well as line managers, including the manager of the newly acquired practice. Frequently, this group must work quickly to transition physicians, support staff, tax identification numbers, vendor agreements, and myriad other elements. The team usually meets weekly during the transition process, which is much more intense than with a new physician start-up.

Communication Matrix

Last, but not least in either priority or implementation, is the issue of communication. Even the potential for change begets rumors—what people don't know, they make up, and it is always worse than reality.

Preparing to communicate about change must start well before that communication is needed. Such preparation includes identifying the audiences, or stakeholders, who will have an interest in the change and the questions or concerns each audience will likely want answered. Each question or concern then needs to be considered and a draft response developed that is consistent with information currently available.

Communication of those responses includes the medium (more likely multimedia), the person responsible for the communication, and a due date. All of these factors are considered in the communication matrix illustrated in Appendix F.

Summary

The role of market manager is critical to the success of all physician-hospital integration efforts, particularly initiatives involving employed physicians. The market manager is ultimately accountable to ensure the development of a primary care retail strategy that drives the development of the physician network. She must also ensure that PCPs (both employed and independent) are connected with specialists of choice and the hospital of choice, both of which can and do attract patient referrals based on top-quality service to referring physicians and their patients.

The wise market manager also ensures that her physician network development efforts are supported by an effective and efficient physician recruitment and practice acquisition engine. She recognizes that in today's highly competitive markets she cannot leave physician network development or relationship management to chance, but must remain actively involved in building, maintaining, and monitoring relationships and performance all along the demand chain for both employed and independent physicians.

References

1. P.F. Drucker, *The Essential Drucker* (New York: HarperCollins, 2001).
2. M. Halley, "The Case for a Medical Practice Retail Strategy," *Journal of Medical Practice Management* November/December (2004): 163–166.
3. K. Cohn and D. Hough, eds., *Practice Management,* 48–50, vol. 1, *The Business of Healthcare* (Westport, CT: Praeger, 2008).
4. M. Halley, *The Primary Care–Market Share Connection: How Hospitals Achieve Competitive Advantage,* 97–111 (Chicago: Health Administration Press, 2007).
5. Ibid., 120–121.
6. Ibid., 120–130.
7. Merritt Hawkins, "2007 Physician Inpatient/Outpatient Revenue Survey" (2008) [www.merritthawkins.com/pdf/2007_Physician_Inpatient_Outpatient_Revenue_Survey.pdf]. Accessed July 19, 2010.
8. Ibid. (2004 data as reported in the 2007 survey results).
9. Merritt Hawkins, "Summary Report: 2005 Survey of Hospital Physician Recruitment Trends" (2005) [www.merritthawkins.com/pdf/mha2005recruitsurvey.pdf]. Accessed July 19, 2010.
10. Cejka Search and American Medical Group Association, *Cejka Search/AMGA 2008 Physician Retention Survey* (Alexandria, VA: American Medical Group Association, 2009). Copyright © 2009, American Medical Group Association. www.amga.org. Used with permission.

CHAPTER 6

Practice and Network Marketing

When interviewing physicians whose hospital-owned practices are not performing well, we often hear concerns that the hospital has not provided enough marketing for the practice. These "marketing" concerns usually relate to inadequate advertising or other means of practice promotion. Sometimes our physician interviewees suggest more newspaper promotion, a larger advertisement in the Yellow Pages, a direct mail campaign, or even billboard advertising. Some hospital executives, on the other hand, feel that their employed physicians are not properly motivated to build their practices. In most cased, both perspectives are partly true. In this chapter we focus on practice promotion. In chapter 7 we discuss motivating physicians to build their practice.

With some notable exceptions, hospitals and health systems in most markets are not known for their marketing prowess. Until the mid-1980s, most hospitals depended on the "build it and they will come" method to attract market share. They employed workshop strategies, building facilities and adding equipment to create a high-tech image that would attract physicians and their patients.[1]

When these strategies became the "minimum ante" to remain competitive, many successful hospitals moved to service line strategies to differentiate themselves from the competition. These centers of excellence helped to define the image of some hospitals in some competitive markets—particularly in those states where certificate-of-need requirements restricted the also-rans. However, in most communities, multiple hospitals developed heart programs, cancer centers, birthing centers, and more, making it difficult to distinguish one from the other *for anyone who cared to notice.*

During recent years, in an effort to use clinical quality as a differentiator, many hospitals have pursued and been awarded "top 100" status. Banners have been hung and promotional materials developed to let the community know about these honors, most of which are legitimate. Some hospitals use public relations techniques to build a community image and then leverage that image with branding campaigns. Still, much of the marketing and promotion that occurs in the industry is relatively unsophisticated.

Categories of Marketing

What does marketing mean for a hospital-owned medical practice network? The answer lies in the traditional definition of the term *marketing*. Marketing and its implementation in successful medical practices are traditionally divided into the following categories:

- Market research
- Product and service development
- Service pricing
- Service promotion and sales
- Service delivery

Market Research

Market research involves understanding the medical practice's customers and their *needs, wants, and priorities* (NWPs). If I am a primary care physician (PCP), my most important customers are women, who make the majority of health care decisions for the family. If I track my new patient referrals, I will likely find that the majority of my new patients come from established patient referrals (word of mouth). If I practice in an urban or suburban area, I will likely find that more than half of my patients live within a short drive of my practice.

If I am a specialty physician and largely dependent on referrals from other physicians and providers, my most important customer is the referring physician, who will diagnose and refer even more patients if I meet the NWPs of that referring physician and his patients.

Product and Service Development

Development of products and services to meet the NWPs of my customers should flow from market research. Service development in a medical practice includes the *types* of services I provide (including the often hotly contested ancillary services), *where* I provide them, *when* I provide them, *how* I package them, and more. The days and hours I am available as well as my scheduling approach are important parts of service development. The payers I accept in my practice are also a part of my service development package.

Service Pricing

Pricing is a traditional aspect of the marketing topic. Pricing in health care has not been a significant source of differentiation in the past, because patients have a difficult time making value/cost comparisons. Those few notable exceptions to this norm include the fee for normal labor and delivery, a sports physical, or a flu shot. However, in general, most of us cannot pronounce the names of most cognitive or surgical medical services, let alone price shop for them.

Service Promotion and Sales

Promotion and *sales* are terms most people associate with marketing. Traditional product or service promotion includes advertising in all its forms, such as newspaper ads, signage, brochures, direct mail, billboards, radio and television spots, Web pages, and Internet pop-up ads. Self-promotion also includes personal interviews, educational presentations, writing for publication, memberships, and so forth.

The sales process involves promoting the product or service but goes well beyond simply delivering a message. Sales includes building a relationship, understanding potential NWPs, matching NWPs to the products and services offered, overcoming customer objections to the terms of the deal, closing the deal, and ensuring effective delivery. In the future, sales will become an increasingly critical part of health care marketing, especially for hospitals and specialty medical practices.

Service Delivery

Service delivery, particularly in a referral-dependent business like medical care, is a significant part of the marketing process. Most primary care practices are dependent on word-of-mouth referrals from existing patients to their friends and neighbors. Specialty physicians are dependent on referrals from PCPs. Both types of referrals are based on relationships, and referral paths are maintained by meeting patient and referring physician NWPs.

The "service experience" is the greatest determinant of continued referrals. That experience has relatively little to do with the clinical competence of the provider(s). Instead, it is largely dependent on how well the customer's service expectations were met, whether that customer be the patient or the patient's referring physician. More on service delivery is offered later in this chapter.

Asking "Who Cares?"

Say I drive through a community near my hometown and notice a sign prominently advertising an "open MRI." I wonder how many of the hundreds of people who pass along that busy highway understand what an open MRI (magnetic resonance imaging machine) is—or even care—let alone know when they need one.

The most important question to answer in deciding what products and services to promote, to whom they should be promoted, and how to promote them is "Who cares?" For example, most of the educated population may have a vague understanding of an MRI as a special kind of "x-ray" machine. They may even know the term *magnetic resonance imaging* from listening to some health care drama or sitcom. But who really cares about that open MRI? The following parties come to mind:

- The owners of the open MRI, some of whom may be physicians
- Referring physicians, as an alternative for their patients who are uncomfortable in closed spaces
- Patients who are (1) told they need an MRI by a physician; (2) claustrophobic and express that fear to their doctor; (3) candidates for an open MRI, given the recommended diagnostic procedure; and (4) educated by their physician, the Internet, or others about the availability of open magnetic resonance imaging

Most of the rest of us really do not care about that open MRI, and efforts to promote the service to us are at least unnecessary and at most an irritant (adding to the clutter of messages already vying for our attention).

Asking "Who cares?" when planning promotional activities will help ensure that the right message reaches the right audience in the right way and at the right time. So who does care about medical services, and what specifically do they care about?

While exceptions certainly exist, when Mrs. Smith asks Mrs. Jones where she takes her children for routine medical services, Mrs. Jones is likely to provide a reference to her own physician. She will most likely refer to that physician by name rather than by the physician's group practice or clinic name or the hospital with which he is affiliated.

When a new primary care physician needs to order an ear, nose, and throat (ENT) consult, he is likely to ask a physician partner whom she refers to for ENT services. The partner is likely to provide a specific ENT's name rather than his group affiliation—although the partner may note that the ENT's group includes several trustworthy doctors.

Many patients do not worry about a physician's hospital affiliation(s) until they need a hospital. (Some women choosing an obstetrician "shop" labor and delivery rooms and select an obstetrician/gynecologist who delivers at their preferred hospital, but this behavior is the exception.)

The hospital's brand can be a real asset to an affiliated medical practice, but it is not likely to come up in the patient-to-patient referral discussion. It may come up in the physician-to-physician discussion, especially when employed physician referrals are tracked. Consequently, medical practice promotional activities for patients, such as the signage, patient statements, direct mail, and so forth, should emphasize first and foremost the physician's name, followed by the group name (if applicable), followed by the employed physician's hospital affiliation.

Should a hospital-owned medical practice network have its own brand? Again, the question is "Who cares?" Most patients do not care because they will not utilize the network of practices. Specialty physicians may care because of the potential referrals coming from multiple PCPs located in multiple neighborhoods—although their referral relationships will be with individual physicians.

The real audience for a network brand is the local payer community. If insurance executives are thinking clearly, they realize that a hospital's affiliated primary care practices hold the payer's current and potential market share, as well. The value of a properly distributed primary care network is (or should be) significant to all those who deal with that network, because those practices hold that market share and direct patient referrals downstream. Insurers will also realize the value of employed specialty physicians and the services they offer, often in concert with hospitals. Selling a hospital-owned network's strengths to selected payers can be a real boon to the integrated system, especially if the employed physician network is substantial enough to command the payer's attention in the local market.

Understanding Needs, Wants, and Priorities

Simply stated, the customers' needs, wants, and priorities should drive organizations' marketing decisions. All three words are important, but particularly so are the wants and priorities. Unfortunately, most medical practices (both primary care and specialty practices) are geared toward meeting the patient's clinical needs.

Let's return to Mrs. Smith and define her NWPs. Imagine a strep (*Streptococcus*) outbreak at the local elementary school. Junior shows up at the school nurse's office at midday with a sore throat. The school nurse is likely to call "Mom." In most communities, Mom is likely to be at work when that call arrives. Given the circumstances, what are Mom's NWPs? The clinical need is a strep test to determine whether Junior has the illness and a note from the doctor as to whether Junior can return to school. But what about Mom's wants?

Mom's wants tend to relate to access. She wants to call her physician and have the phone answered immediately. She wants to get an appointment for Junior today. She wants that appointment to be with her preferred doctor. She wants to feel valued by the receptionist, the nurse, and the physician. She wants a short wait time in the reception room and the examination room. She wants the ancillary services readily available in her doctor's office. She wants an antibiotic to validate her reason for the office visit.

Finally, what about her priorities? Mrs. Smith's priorities relate to her own life (her challenges, commitments, roles, responsibilities, and schedule) rather than her doctor's office. Her ultimate priority is Junior, but that ultimate priority must be balanced by the fact that she has a sales presentation at a luncheon meeting with clients from 11:45 AM until 1:30 PM. It is also her day to take the neighborhood children to soccer practice at 4:45 PM. The commute to the school is twenty minutes; she will spend ten minutes to check Junior out of school and eight minutes to get to the doctor's office. Based on these priorities, she requires an appointment after 2:00 PM and must leave the doctor's no later than 4:15 PM so Junior can dress and have a snack before practice, which he refuses to miss. Unrealistic? Not at all.

Mrs. Smith can get a strep test and a doctor's note from several places, including the local urgent care, the local Walgreens pharmacy, the nearby Wal-Mart store, or the local grocery. If the doctor's office cannot or chooses not to meet Mrs. Smith's wants and priorities, she will be forced to go elsewhere today—and perhaps forevermore.

What about the specialty physician's most important customer? Understanding and meeting referring physician NWPs are critical to maintaining referral relationships, which are increasingly vulnerable today. Based on discussions, interviews, and surveys conducted by The Halley Consulting Group, the most significant NWPs for referring physicians and other providers are the following:

- *Access.* Access to specialists is the number one NWP expressed by referring physicians. Access includes the ability to schedule patients in a timely manner and assurance of specialist participation in insurance plans used by the PCPs' patients. Access sometimes means showing up in satellite settings to serve the patients in rural areas; it also includes the specialist's willingness to take Medicaid and uninsured patients as well as those with better insurance coverage. Few situations are more frustrating to referring physicians than encountering specialists who "cherry pick" only those patients with good health insurance.
- *Communication.* Referring physicians want to be able to count on appropriate feedback from specialists to whom they refer patients. *Appropriate* is the key word that separates preferred specialists from those who will be replaced as soon as an alternative becomes available. Some referring physicians prefer to visit with the specialist before the consultation takes place in order to discuss the PCP's objectives for the visit/consult. Other PCPs do not require communication until the specialist has seen the patient. Many referring physicians would like to be involved in the discussion of the initial diagnosis and the treatment plan proposed by the specialist. Others want the specialist to perform her service and provide feedback after the visit. Some referring physicians prefer to communicate by telephone; others are comfortable with e-mail or with the traditional letter from the specialist. How does a specialist know the preferences of referring physicians? He asks those he wants to keep and records their preferences in a profile that is accessed by his staff members every time a referral is received. That profile is updated periodically by physician liaisons employed at the hospital or by the specialist herself as she visits with each PCP.
- *Service quality.* The experience of referred patients will most certainly make its way back to the referring physician. This factor relates to "how I felt I was treated" rather than the clinical outcome. Patients who are delighted with their service experience at the specialty office will report

> that experience to their "regular doctor." Specialists and their office staff members who do not provide a great service experience to each patient create a problem for the referring physician—the death knell for future referrals if an alternative is available.

Many specialists will ask "What about the role of clinical quality?" Interestingly, as mentioned in chapter 5, clinical quality is not usually listed among the top motivating factors for referring physicians. When we inquire as to the reason for this apparent oversight, the referring physicians almost always respond that clinical quality is assumed. Clinical quality affects the referral decision when it is *not* present.

Practice Evolution

The challenge of meeting the NWPs of Mrs. Smith seems manageable when the practice is small. It can provide access, it has time to "be nice," and the doctor can take time for the secondary (or tertiary) clinical issue or the social conversation that often follows the chief complaint in the examination room. However, as the practice becomes busier, the reception desk is bombarded with phone calls as the receptionist tries to check in six patients an hour instead of the previous three, and verifying insurance information and collecting co-payments in the process. Errors increase, causing rework at the front desk, the nurse's station, and the cashier's window, not to mention the billing office. The reception room becomes a waiting room because the doctor is constantly running behind schedule. The nurse is rushed trying to keep three examination rooms full, responding to the physician's needs and instructions, drawing blood and giving injections—all while fighting with insurance carriers for pre-authorizations, calling in approved prescription refills, and trying to get a Medicaid patient scheduled with a specialist. The physician is frustrated at his inability to keep up as the hours he spends each day stretch into the evenings. Most importantly, the patients *feel* the rushed atmosphere. They struggle to get an appointment, they have to wait too long, and they feel like the doctor does not listen anymore. As a result, Mrs. Smith may now be less inclined to give a glowing report or to refer the doctor at all.

Meeting the NWPs of referring physicians is an equally daunting challenge faced by most successful physician specialists. Let's again consider the common evolution of a new specialty practice.

A new specialist, Dr. Jones, starts practice in the community. The traditional newspaper announcements are followed by personal visits to meet and distribute business cards to potential referring physicians. During the second week of practice, Dr. Jones receives his first referral from Dr. Case. Dr. Jones personally takes the call from Dr. Case to discuss the situation and immediately schedules the patient for a consultation. After the examination, Dr. Jones quickly contacts

Dr. Case to personally discuss the findings and treatment plan. This personal interaction is followed by an eight-page letter providing a thorough explanation of findings, diagnosis, and treatment. The letter closes with sincere thanks from Dr. Jones for the referral. The patient is returned to Dr. Case for follow-up, where she reports that Dr. Jones and his staff are wonderful. Dr. Case looks like a hero for referring to Dr. Jones, and she determines to try the specialist again.

This scenario is repeated for several referring physicians over the next few months. Referrals continue to grow, and the volume of consults and procedures soon begins to stretch Dr. Jones and his support staff. Before long, Dr. Jones is so busy that he cannot often get to the phone when a referring physician calls because he is in the examination room or in the operating room. His office visits are shorter than they had been previously, and his letters to referring physicians barely reach two pages and contain just the clinical essentials, using stock paragraphs. He scrambles to return phone calls from physicians, patients, and others within the same day. Dr. Jones' support staff members are feeling the pressure, as well. They are so busy trying to keep up that the customer (the patient or the referring physician) experience becomes secondary to surviving the day.

The volume of patient referrals coming as a result of easy access, rapid and thorough communication, and a great patient experience is now choking Dr. Jones' practice. Referral relationships have become vulnerable to astute competitors who can better manage their success.

As stated earlier, every decision, policy, procedure, process, form, design, and activity in an individual medical practice or in a large network of practices must pass the following four critical success filters:

1. Does it maintain or enhance clinical quality as defined by our physicians?
2. Does it maintain or enhance service quality as defined by our patients and their referring physicians?
3. Does it maintain physician productivity (the key to maintaining service levels and revenue)?
4. Does it maintain practice operational and financial viability?

These four filters are the essence of marketing a medical practice, which ultimately grows (despite newspaper ads, direct mail, and billboards) as a result of referrals from satisfied patients and satisfied referring physicians.

Customer Service—the Ultimate Marketing Tool

Combine a bright young physician, a great support staff, word-of-mouth referrals from happy patients, and enough referring physicians, and success is inevitable. So, it appears, is the challenge of remaining accessible and responsive when that success occurs. As I have written in the past, *referrals follow relationships*, and *all relationships atrophy over time.*[2] Managing the patient experience and those referral relationships for the long term requires more than just being nice and working harder and longer. Maintaining access, effective communication, and a great patient experience in the face of tremendous success requires proper support staffing, effective job design, efficient internal systems, streamlined processes, customer-oriented policies, and even employee scripting. Success requires that the physician learn to practice more efficiently while maintaining his or her effectiveness. Maintaining relationships certainly requires careful monitoring and service recovery when errors or problems are detected.

The busiest successful practices tend to have more full-time-equivalent staff members per physician than do their less successful counterparts. They are not overstaffed; they are properly and adequately staffed to maximize productivity and minimize distractions for the three primary roles in a medical practice: the physician (or mid-level provider), the clinical assistant, and the receptionist. All other roles are secondary and exist to support the primary roles. We discuss staffing and productivity, including the concepts of highest and best-use staffing[3] and job design, in chapter 8.

Retail Readiness

Retail readiness[4] is composed of the critical processes that make or break a growing practice. They include the following components:

1. The referral
2. The initial contact
3. The appointment desk
4. The reception
5. Waiting
6. The clinical assistant
7. The physician visit
8. The close
9. Billing and collections
10. The next referral

Let's examine each process with the patient/customer in mind whom you wish to retain.

The Referral

Those people receiving services and those providing services are all dependent, at one time or another, on a referral from someone else. The new primary care patient usually receives a referral from a friend to help select a PCP. The PCP's practice grows largely through word of mouth from existing patients, who become a passive sales force.[5] When the patient needs a specialty referral, the PCP is most likely to make that referral, as the patient does not usually know when a specialty visit is indicated or which specialist to see. The specialist is dependent on the PCP to refer patients, and those referrals are built on the kinds of relationships previously discussed. With the exception of the emergency department, most other hospital services are dependent on referrals directly from PCPs or indirectly from PCPs through specialists.

Each referral comes with an implied promise from the referrer that the referent physician or hospital department will meet the customer's NWPs. This promise creates a set of expectations in the mind of the customer relative to his or her NWPs. It is now up to the specialist and support staff, or the hospital department staff and hospital-based physicians, to meet those expectations. The challenge is to send every customer away saying "Wow, what a great experience!" In fact, we often us the concept of wow factors when we work with physicians and their staff members to improve their service outcomes.

The Initial Contact

The first impression sets the tone for the service experience. Common wow factors for patients include a human being answering the phone who is obviously delighted that the patient called.

We hear all kinds of arguments about reducing labor costs and increasing productivity. These points are certainly valid, but they do not pass all four critical success filters. Even in today's high-tech world, most customers prefer to be greeted by a human. As volume increases, additional task specialization is required (a topic we further discuss in chapter 8). Employing a switchboard operator (or two during the busiest times) will help ensure that our patients' expectations are met.

Referring physicians, of course, should have their own back line that is always answered promptly by a competent and scripted staff member: "Dr. Case, I know that Dr. Jones will want to speak with you. He is in an exam room with a patient right now. Would you like me to interrupt him?" The usual answer is "no." The script continues: "Where can Dr. Jones reach you in the next twenty minutes?" The number is taken and immediately handed to Dr. Jones' clinical assistant, who gets Dr. Case on the phone as Dr. Jones moves between exam rooms. Impossible? Not if adequate staff are available and doing just the right things.

The Appointment Desk

The appointment desk is the acid test for busy practices. What wows patients? Having the practice meet the patient's first or second request for an appointment time. How often does this happen? The practice should know the answer each day. If a caller cannot get in to see "my doctor" today, is he offered acceptable alternatives such as a competent partner or a mid-level provider, or is his best alternative going to the local Wal-Mart in-store clinic for care? Certainly, individual physicians have limits, as do group practices, but no legitimate patient should be turned away. (Drug seekers and those who refuse to pay their bills would not be considered legitimate customers.)

Some practices offer extended hours for their patients. Some use open-access scheduling models to see all patients the same day. Others provide a nurse practitioner or physician assistant as an alternative. (Most mid-level providers build their own patient base over time, but in our experience they rarely fill up completely.) Some practices use the first- or second-request indicator to determine when to add another partner. As a last resort, some will transfer a patient to another practice within the medical practice network.

The Reception

How are patients greeted when they enter the office? Do they stare through bulletproof glass at emotionless staff sitting behind the protective cover, or are they warmly greeted by a smiling receptionist who acts as if she has been waiting to call them by name and welcome them to the practice?

Is the receptionist more concerned about the patient's insurance card or about making the customer feel welcome? The right receptionist with the right personality and the right training on the right practice management system can verify insurance information, ask for co-payment, greet the patient who follows, invite the patient to be comfortably seated, and still make her "glad I came today." To achieve this wow standard, any nonrelated responsibilities must be removed from the front desk and given to someone in a secondary role.

Waiting

A waiting room is like a black hole. There is a way in, but the way out is unclear. The patient has been checked in by the front desk, filled out paperwork, shared insurance information, and watched as the glass window is closed. The customer is no longer the front desk's responsibility, but she is not yet the nurse's responsibility.

A reception room, on the other hand, is comfortable and is staffed by an attentive receptionist who remains aware of each patient and how long he or she has been waiting. In fact, she is scripted to express the doctor's concern if the doctor is running late and to ask if the patient is still able to wait. The receptionist is like a lifeguard watching for discontent and practicing scripted service recovery if necessary. The patient is kept informed and comfortable, remaining in the receptionist's capable hands until called back by the clinical assistant.

Waiting, of course, in all its forms is the enemy of a positive service experience and must be prevented (through appropriate scheduling, provider productivity, etc.) or overcome by acknowledgment and apology.

The Clinical Assistant

The clinical assistant has two very important roles in the medical practice: to ensure that the patient has a positive experience from a clinical and service perspective and to drive physician productivity. The second role is discussed in the "Practice Operations Management" section of chapter 8.

The first responsibility commences when the patient is personally called from the reception room and warmly greeted. The arrival time and appointment time are noted on the chart, so the clinical assistant can apologize if that time spread exceeds the practice's service commitment.

In most traditional settings, the clinical assistant records the patient's weight and accompanies her to an examination room, where they discuss the chief complaint and at which time the patient's vital signs are taken. The clinical assistant helps the patient prepare for the physician's examination, including offering a cloth gown and even a warm blanket if disrobing is necessary. The clinical assistant periodically checks on the patient—tapping on the door each time before entering the room—and keeps her informed as to her place in the queue. The assistant may or may not be present during the doctor's examination but is always present at the exam's conclusion.

As the physician departs, the clinical assistant receives any instructions to obtain specimens and to close the visit. The handoff is comfortable because the patient is familiar with the clinical assistant who initiated the visit.

The Physician Visit

Several practice-related events have already taken place before the patient sees the physician. Those events have either placed the physician on a pedestal or dug a hole so deep that she may never crawl out. The well-scripted physician notes the appointment time and apologizes if service commitments have not been met. The most important service commitment by the physician is to listen, listen, and listen.

From the patient's perspective, they are gathered here to talk about *him*—his feelings, his ills, his concerns. He is not a lab rat or a "diagnosis." What the physician knows is important, but not as important as the patient's feeling that he and his issues are the main focus, regardless of how many cases the doctor has already seen of this virus today and that the patient could have been diagnosed from the hallway. Importantly, the physician should always compliment the patient for coming in today, thus validating the decision to do so.

To be most effective, the physician must quickly assess the patient's personality and respond within that context. If the patient is in the examination room with his mother, the doctor must assess both personalities and respond appropriately. Does the patient expect straightforward information? If the patient is a child, is the physician expected to caress his head while you talk with the mother? Is a little light-hearted joke warranted?

It is always profitable to acknowledge the good work of your clinical assistant as you assess the information provided through the workup. She will be the person to whom the physician hands off the patient at the end of the visit; the expressed confidence in her will increase the patient's level of confidence in her.

Obviously, somewhere in the midst of the service experience in the examination room, the physician must conduct a physical examination, determine a diagnosis, identify the treatment, and communicate the findings in clear and understandable language.

The Close

Ideally, as the physician completes her work in the examination room, the clinical assistant is right at the door waiting for a smooth handoff. She receives the doctor's instructions in the patient's presence. In the process, the physician compliments both of the others where possible. The assistant then completes the clinical process by reiterating critical instructions and asking if the patient has any additional questions. If a specialty referral or ancillary services are necessary (at any time during or after the visit) the clinical assistant provides direction and support to the patient. Like the physician, the clinical assistant sincerely thanks the patient for coming and accompanies him to the cashier station.

The cashier is the person who talks with the patient about money and insurance questions. His job is to *help the patient* get the physician paid. In the process, he asks about the service experience. He answers financial questions. He asks if the patient needs to make another appointment and either makes that appointment on the spot or smoothly transitions the patient to the appointment specialist.

Billing and Collections

"How can we help you get us paid?" That question sets the tone for customer-oriented billing and collections. The most successful processes we have experienced have this philosophy at their core. The physician practice is on the same side of the table as its customer. It is his advocate—even if the patient does not have insurance or his insurance reimburses poorly. The practice is always prepared to "go to bat" for its customers with their carriers. Its staff are happy to answer their insurance questions, to provide updates on payments, and to file secondary claims.

Patient statements are clear and easy to understand because staff have looked at them from the vantage point of the customer. The practice handles billing calls in the clinic site as well as in the central processing office. It provides payment plans and offers options to those who need charity care. The practice will dismiss patients who do not take responsibility for their balances due, but it is with regret that this action is taken, and it is taken only after the office manager has personally tried to work with them.

The Next Referral

We are back to the beginning of the process. Has each service experience wowed the patients? Will they naturally and comfortably risk referring the practice to their friends and relatives?

Becoming the Specialist of Choice

How do physicians earn a reputation as the specialist of choice?[6] In other words, when a new PCP moves to town and joins a small group practice, how does he choose which specialists to use for consults? Does he review the morbidity, mortality, or other quality statistics increasingly available for specialty services? Unlikely. In actuality, the new physician does what Mrs. Smith does when she moves to town: He asks a neighbor, in this case a partner: "To whom do you refer for a cardiology consult?" Of course, the experienced physician partner has completed the required research and directs his new partner to the most proficient cardiologist in town, right? Wrong. He directs the new partner to the cardiologist with whom he has a satisfactory referral relationship. That relationship, as we have discussed, is based on factors such as access, communication, and patient experience.

As indicated earlier, becoming the specialist of choice involves a clear understanding of two very important factors:[7]

- Referrals follow relationships.
- All relationships atrophy over time.

Those of us who watch and promote changes in market share, as well as those who have been the victims of those changes, realize just how vulnerable are professional referral relationships. A friendship struck over dinner between an internist and a new surgeon yields referrals from the internist regardless of past relationships. A memorandum from the hospital chief executive officer to employed referring physicians requiring them to "refer domestic" (refer only to affiliated specialists and hospitals) quickly changes referral patterns. Access problems force a referring physician to try another specialist or group, and a new relationship is born.

On one occasion we were asked to assess why a network of employed physicians was referring its patients to non-affiliated physicians and services—specifically radiology services. I found the answer in the first interview. The family physician said: "I call our radiology department to schedule a mammogram, and it is at least a one-week wait. I call the group down the street at the competing hospital, and they commit to see the patient within forty-eight hours—and they act like they want my business!" So much for the concept of specialists of choice.

The specialist-of-choice practice evaluation presented in Appendix G includes fifty questions in the following six categories:

1. Referral source knowledge (questions 1–5)
2. Referral source access (questions 6–21)
3. Referral source expectations (questions 22–25)
4. Customer service team (questions 26–32)
5. Relationship management (questions 33–47)
6. Education/promotion (questions 48–50)

While this self-evaluation is generic, the questions should prompt appropriate customer-oriented thought processes for any single-specialty practice or multispecialty department. We recommend that the physicians, mid-level providers, support staff members, and management team meet quarterly to complete the questionnaire. In addition, we recommend that they select two items per quarter to improve upon and establish tactics, performance targets, performance measures, and timelines and assign responsibility for completing tactics.

Again, the concept of wow factors is relevant as we consider what would wow or amaze our referring physicians and their clinical assistants or referral coordinators as they deal with our specialty practice. Certain tactics can even become service commitments that the practice makes public. Service commitments can be developed and implemented by hospital service line, engaging physicians and hospital departments in identifying the NWPs of referring physicians and their patients, developing commitments around those NWPs, and then rigorously measuring and consistently meeting those commitments. Performance measures should be reviewed at least monthly to determine whether performance is adequate and progress is being made.

Other Promotional Techniques—Primary Care

When establishing promotional tactics for primary care and specialty medical practices, we return to the concept of "Who cares?" Techniques we have successfully used in primary care practices include the following:

- Newspaper announcements
- Direct mail

- Telephone book listings
- Community education
- Web page development

Newspaper Announcements

The traditional newspaper announcement is a "shotgun" approach that ignores the fact that the majority of patients living in urban or suburban settings will select a PCP close to home. Further, of those patients who see the physician's advertisement, the majority will not be motivated to act because they do not need a physician right now—or they are already attached to another PCP. Some may be motivated to clip the ad and remember the new physician, but these will likely be very few.

Still, newspaper advertising is a relatively inexpensive way to reach many households and is more important as a promotional tool in smaller communities, where a weekly paper contains many significant announcements for the smaller populous. We have found that newspaper ads featuring a nice picture of a photogenic physician seem to increase the numbers of potential patients who take action. We have also found that ads that go beyond mentioning board certification, which most people do not understand, and include the physician's special clinical interests are more likely to motivate action. For example, an advertisement indicating that the physician has a special interest or training in headaches or sleep disorders seems to immediately attract calls from those who relate to these maladies.

Direct Mail

We always recommend the development of a promotional sheet for new and established physicians. The promotional sheet usually includes a nice picture of the physician and a biographical sketch that includes education, certifications, and special clinical interests. Some physicians prefer to include a bit of personal information, such as hobbies or a meaningful quote. These sheets are professionally produced on glossy paper and can be used as direct mail pieces targeted to the practice neighborhood (usually within a ten-minute drive in urban and suburban areas). Some communities have direct mail services that hand-deliver these pieces for a nominal fee. Other practices choose to develop the sheets with mailing information on the reverse side. We have found that direct mail yields new patients who live within the neighborhood.

Telephone Book Listings

Telephone books continue to be an important source for patients trying to locate a practice or physician. Primary care practices still encounter patients who have selected the physician by consulting the Yellow Pages. Whether they are looking for a location near home or are attracted by quarter-page ads is still not documented. Regardless, the telephone directory continues to be an important promotional tool.

Community Education

Positioning oneself as the expert on a topic of interest to potential patients or referral sources is a proven way to attract additional referrals. That positioning can occur in several different ways, including the following:

- *Mass media*. Some hospitals have speakers bureaus that offer physician experts as a community resource to address specific topics. Radio and television news spots often include health care topics, and an articulate physician can be positioned as a local expert to address issues specific to her specialty. Journalists are often looking for experts to quote for local news articles, which again positions the physician nicely in the local environment.
- *Health fairs*. Community service health fairs are a potential source of new business, particularly for primary care specialties. Providing meaningful information and simple screening tests can introduce physicians and staff members to the community.
- *Neighborhood locations*. A powerful neighborhood strategy for PCPs includes targeting specific groups of people and providing education on topics of interest. For example, schools, nursing homes, day care centers, church gatherings, clubs, and other groups often provide a willing audience whose members will benefit from attending. Health care topics usually generate interest and can be crafted to the audience in terms of age and gender issues. Having a day care center offer a visit with a local physician as a service to parents benefits the day care center, the parents, the children, and the physician. Practice managers are often a great resource to identify and approach these groups to solicit interest.

Web Page Development

Technology is an increasingly important part of our daily lives. Many people routinely use the Internet to conduct research, catch up with old friends, express opinions, and purchase all kinds of goods and services. The Web can also be a great place for medical practices to address an increasing number of patients. Some medical practices allow their patients to schedule appointments, check laboratory results, review practice policies, and post questions for the physician(s) via a Web portal. While a Web site is a potentially potent promotional tool and patient resource, it does require maintenance to remain effective.

A variety of other techniques and tools may be used by PCPs to promote their practices, ranging from refrigerator magnets to open houses and beyond. It is critical to remember, even in this high-tech society, that the most reliable means of building a primary care practice is through word of mouth from customers based on a great service experience.

Other Promotional Techniques—Specialty Practices

The introduction of hospitalists has a number of benefits in local markets. One downside of this trend is that far fewer PCPs conduct rounds in hospitals, where they encounter specialists in the hallways or medical staff lounge. Some busy PCPs are opting to avoid medical staff meetings and even reconsidering medical staff membership and the requirements for meeting attendance, on-call coverage, and so forth. This trend presents a significant challenge for specialty physicians who may rarely or never see a referring physician face-to-face.

Promotional activities for specialists vary. Surgeons would not benefit much, even if they could attract an audience, by sharing the latest laparoscopic techniques at an elementary school parent-teacher association meeting. They might, however, benefit from sharing those same techniques in a medical staff newsletter or hospital-sponsored town hall meeting that reaches a PCP audience. Those specialties with a large number of patient self-referrals (e.g., dermatology) would benefit from mirroring several primary care promotional techniques. Those without many self-referrals need to reach the audience that guides those referral decisions.

When a new invasive specialty physician moves to town, the traditional newspaper announcements alert the population and the medical staff that she is available for consultation. The population will not likely care because they do not know when a surgeon is indicated. The medical staff may care, especially if the new specialist is desperately needed in the community. We usually recommend that hospitals create a nice, formal announcement to the medical staff and medical community at large that shares the new physician's credentials, experience, and contact information. This mailer may be accompanied by a business card. We also recommend the development of professional-looking service sheets describing certain ailments routinely managed by the specialist and make them available to PCPs as education pieces for their patients. Of course, each service sheet has information on the backside describing the specialty practice, including a map of its location.

Next to a referral from an established PCP to a new physician partner, the most powerful promotional tool for new specialists is initiating a personal relationship with potential referring physicians. In the early days of practice, while a new specialist has extra time available, she should be out meeting PCPs and other referral sources. These meetings can be arranged by the specialist's office manager or a hospital-employed physician liaison. They might be as simple as a brief introduction and exchange of business cards or might extend to an offer to bring a light lunch for the PCP and staff. Dinner meetings between primary care and specialty groups previously unknown to one another are an excellent way for hospitals to promote new referrals to both new and established practices. Once these relationships are initiated, it is up to the specialist and her support staff to remain the specialist of choice.

Summary

The days of "hanging out a shingle" and waiting for a medical practice to prosper are long gone. While the tools of medical practice promotion need not be sophisticated, understanding the varied needs, wants, and priorities of customer segments requires increasing attention and expertise. So does building practice policies, procedures, training, and culture around customer service. Most practices and hospitals are still largely dependent on word-of-mouth referrals from satisfied patients and satisfied referring physicians. Satisfied patients build primary care practices. Satisfied PCPs build specialty practices.

Building and maintaining what are increasingly vulnerable relationships is the key to success in competitive markets. The essence of those relationships is a consistently high-quality service experience. Combining that experience with a few well-placed promotional tools ensures the success of a primary care or specialty practice.

References

1. M. Halley, *The Primary Care–Market Share Connection: How Hospitals Achieve Competitive Advantage,* 1–3 (Chicago: Health Administration Press, 2007).
2. Ibid., 120–121.
3. M. Halley and M. Ferry, *The Medical Practice Start-Up Guide,* 72–74 (Phoenix, MD: Greenbranch, 2008).
4. Halley, *The Primary Care–Market Share Connection,* 25–27.
5. Ibid., 38–39.
6. K. Cohn and D. Hough, eds., *Practice Management,* 48–50, vol. 1, *The Business of Healthcare* (Westport, CT: Praeger, 2008).
7. Halley, *The Primary Care–Market Share Connection,* 120–121.

CHAPTER 7

Human Resource Issues

This chapter is intended to highlight only the most common human resource issues faced by hospitals that own medical practices. Readers seeking a more complete explanation of related issues are referred to Halley and Ferry's *The Medical Practice Start-Up Guide*.[1]

Common Profiles: Physician Employees

Physicians are the most highly trained clinicians in the United States. As mentioned in chapter 2, they are Peter Drucker's classic knowledge workers.[2] They own the "means of production" in terms of their knowledge and practiced skills. All have spent years in post–high school and postgraduate education. Their clinical expertise is unquestioned—at least for the majority of their group. They are licensed by the state in which they practice to provide access to legally controlled substances and to perform invasive procedures with full awareness of the attendant risks to human life.

Many physicians are among the brightest of the bright in terms of intellect and among the most highly skilled of technicians. Yet physicians are human beings, subject to all the human frailties and challenges of "lesser mortals." Despite their intellectual prowess, some suffer failing marriages; others struggle with wayward children. Even with their high income potential, most still have to work to meet their mortgage payments. They feel pain, anxiety, and frustration. They become weary and cross. They hope for a better quality of life than their parents or physician predecessors had. Some are mission driven; others are greedy. Some trip over their own pride on occasion. Most physicians are fine people just trying to make it through life, contributing to society where they can.

Common Profiles: Small Group Practice Managers

In a hospital setting, many department managers are at least bachelor's prepared in their area of specialty, and most executives are master's prepared. While larger medical groups often employ managers or administrators with similar credentials to those managing in hospital departments, many small medical office managers do not have academic credentials beyond a high school diploma. In fact, a number of them started out as receptionists or medical assistants in their practices. They are great daily operations people who have received their education on the job.

Those managers who have survived and worked their way to the top are often bright and capable in their own realm. They have followed the direction of the physician-owners and have become effective implementers. However, when brought into a hospital-owned medical practice network, they may shrink at the thought of having bottom line accountability, building a budget, and providing a monthly variance report. They may struggle with the myriad new human resource and other policies. They will likely be confused about surviving in a large bureaucracy. Some will wonder how they relate to their former physician practice owners and to their new "boss," who wears a hospital name tag.

Common Profiles: Support Staff Members

While the physician owns the means of production, the support staff make or break the practice. For example, at least nine "moments of truth"[3] occur before a new patient ever meets a physician for the first time:

1. The referral from a friend or referring physician
2. The phone call for an appointment
3. The search for the office
4. The greeting at the reception desk
5. The new-patient paperwork
6. The reception wait
7. The clinical assistant greeting
8. The chief complaint and patient work-up
9. The exam room wait

Only after these moments of truth does the physician enter the scene. Support staff members control the new patient's experience for the majority of those moments.

A few staff members may have college degrees in nursing or management. Most do not. Many support staff members are wonderful people who view their roles as a *job* rather than a *career*. They want to do well at work, and they enjoy the paycheck and what it allows them to do outside of work. That receptionist who answers the telephone first is probably the lowest-paid person in the practice, but he or she creates an initial impression that clearly reflects on the physician.

As consultants, we have been asked to evaluate primary care practices that were not growing as quickly as anticipated or specialty practices in which specialists were getting negative feedback from referring physicians about access. On more than one occasion, the problem was a receptionist who "wanted" (more likely needed, in order to meet child care or other obligations) to leave work on time and quit taking new appointments after 3:00 PM even though the physician was available and willing to see additional patients.

While admittedly not 100 percent accurate, these employee profiles are reasonably close to reality for most small group medical practices. It is important to remember that joining a large network of hospital-owned practices does not change these small group practice realities. That small practice is still "their" world. The implications of these profiles are significant in terms of motivation, ability, engagement, compensation, employee benefits, training, supervision, and accountability.

Assessing Motivation and Ability

Figure 7-1 illustrates the application of a Johari window to the motivation and ability of human resources in a medical practice (and in any other work situation). A Johari window is a cognitive psychological tool created by Joseph Luft and

Figure 7-1. A Johari Window for Assessing Motivation and Ability

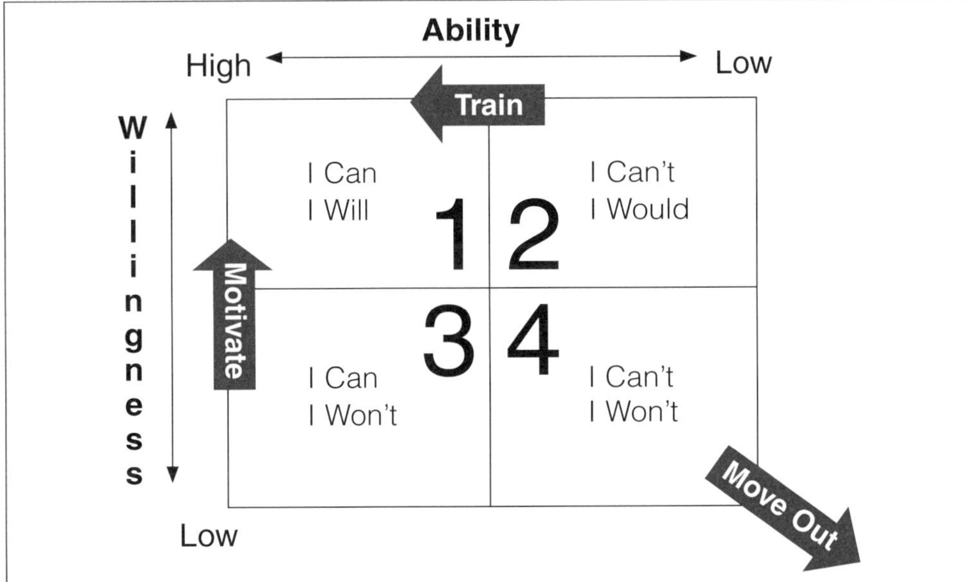

Note: For our purposes, the horizontal axis (x-axis) represents an employee's ability to accomplish his or her work or a particular task. The vertical axis (y-axis) represents an employee's willingness to accomplish his or her work or a particular task. A quadrant 1 employee exhibits high ability and high willingness on the job. A quadrant 2 employee is very willing to serve but lacks the ability to accomplish a task or role within an organization. A quadrant 3 employee has the ability to accomplish a task or an assignment but lacks the willingness to do so. A quadrant 4 employee has neither the ability to perform nor the interest in performing the task or job. Managers can use the Johari window to assess an employee's overall job performance or ability and willingness to perform a specific task.

Source: This Johari window is an adaptation of a matrix that was developed by Joseph Luft and Harry Ingham.

Harry Ingham in 1955. Quadrant 1 includes the names of those individuals who are highly capable and highly motivated. These are the practice's "A players." They can and do accomplish their tasks. They work independently and can be depended on to represent the practice and the physicians well.

Quadrant 2 includes those staff who are highly motivated but not capable of fulfilling their responsibilities. They are solid "B players," who are candidates for additional training to make them A players for the practice.

Quadrant 3 includes employees who are highly skilled but not motivated enough to get the job done. This staff member may need a new opportunity to learn, a new assignment, or other incentives to perform. He or she may require what Frederick W. Herzberg calls a KITA (kick in the "tail").[4] Quadrant 3 players are also B players.

Those staff who fall into quadrant 4 are the highest-risk employees to retain. They have neither the ability nor the interest to contribute to the organization. At best, these "C players" are placeholders—filling a spot, but requiring the support of other team members to perform adequately and frustrating the A players who have to cover for them. At worst, they irreparably damage the reputation and performance of the medical practice. They cannot or refuse to be trained or motivated. They should be replaced, yet we find C players among support staff, management, and even occasionally physicians.

Managers should facilitate the progress of each employee into quadrant 1: Quadrant 2 employees need training and experience; quadrant 3 staff need motivation; quadrant 4 employees need to be moved out of the organization. Thus, facilitating both training and motivation is part of the role of the manager.

Physician and executive leaders on the network operations council (NOC) should ensure that C player physicians and other providers are removed from the practices and the network as a whole. Practice operations councils (POCs) should ensure that B player managers and support staff are trained or motivated and that C players are removed. Small group practices cannot afford to have even one C player among the ranks.

Supervision

Medical practices are labor intensive rather than capital intensive. Although some very sophisticated technology is employed in many medical settings, the provision of medical services to individuals requires people—both knowledge workers and those who support them. The knowledge workers have been trained to provide their services using particular methods and equipment. The support staff must be organized to support those knowledge workers and their methods with processes designed to facilitate the delivery of high-quality care in a caring environment. Such organization requires a clear definition of processes, appropriate definitions of roles and responsibilities, the addition of technology and other equipment where appropriate, the proper use of that technology and equipment (training and ability), and the motivation to perform well. Performance measurement and feedback are critical to ensure that the people, processes, and technology are, indeed, providing the services effectively (delivering the intended services and outcomes) and efficiently (in a resource-conscious manner).

The presence of people in any service delivery process creates variability, not to mention the variety of expectations of the customers (both patients and referring physicians). This potential variability requires constant feedback and process adjustment.

In our experience, ensuring that people, processes, and technology meet the needs, wants, and priorities of our medical practice customers in an effective and efficient manner requires supervision. In solo or very small practices, that supervision may be provided part time by physician-owners. Once a practice has more than a very few employees, all the moving parts require constant oversight. Otherwise, processes and people tend to stray, being influenced by personal preference or objectives, competing physician directives, internal politics, personalities, time off, and many other factors.

Supervision of small group practices and departments in large group practices is an essential part of managing these labor-intensive organizations. For this reason, we recommended the presence of an assigned office manager, who has bottom line accountability, for every practice setting. We also recommend that those managers be present in their assigned practice or practices 95 percent of the time. They have to be present to manage—to provide the required oversight.

Performance Monitoring and Feedback

Monitoring the effectiveness and efficiency of people, processes, and technology in a medical practice setting requires that managers focus some of their attention on the B players. B players are in need of training to improve or expand their abilities and/or motivation to encourage top performance. We recommend the use of the critical incident method[5] of performance appraisal (described below) to ensure ongoing monitoring and performance feedback for individual employees. Because managers are present in their practices, they can personally oversee people and processes on an ongoing basis. They can also solicit feedback from physicians, patients, and support staff peers regarding the effectiveness and efficiency of individuals and processes. Process issues can be addressed in staff meetings and other platforms to be discussed later.

The critical incident method highlights those individual performance issues that vary from expectations—both positive variance and negative variance. Critical incidents are documented by the manager, who then provides timely feedback directly and personally to the individual employee. The employee also receives a copy of the note documenting the incident, and a copy is placed in the employee's personnel file.

Critical incidents provide opportunities for managers to recognize and acknowledge exceptional work as it occurs. They also identify training and motivation issues for individual employees, which become the manager's charge in his or her role to ensure the success of *every willing employee.* Critical incident notes support the formal performance appraisal process by providing situations and examples to support an individual employee's annual performance scores.

Training and Development

"Sharpening the saw" is a matter often ignored in busy organizations, including medical practices and networks. The standard medical practice is so busy that unless managers are diligent, training is permanently sidelined for most support staff, even though the physician fulfills his or her continuing medical education requirements. Training and development are, however, so critical to the short- and long-term success of the organization that they cannot be left to chance. In order to be successful in today's challenging health care environment, every member of the team has to consistently perform at a high level.

Training starts with identifying minimum competencies for each role or job in the organization. Those competencies include the minimum tasks that must be competently performed in order to support clinical quality, service quality, physician productivity, and practice operational and financial viability. The competencies list should inform the employee recruitment process and should be the basis of each new employee orientation. We recommend that the new employee and the supervisor or assigned trainer initial each task on the competency list as it is completed. Ideally, the employee should wear a "trainee" badge until the competencies are attained, to encourage customers to be patient.

In addition to support staff members meeting minimum competencies, POCs and their practice managers should ensure that periodic training occurs for each employee. Training is an investment that motivates employees and emphasizes the importance of quality performance. Training may be job or role specific, such as an update on procedure coding, or it may be general in nature, such as a customer service primer. The manager should ensure that every employee has a POC-approved opportunity to continue learning and developing skills. Training forums may include:

- *Seminars.* Professional associations frequently offer training opportunities to their members. Membership and participation help both clinical and business support staff members "sharpen the saw" and should be pursued at least annually. Attendance also allows participants to interact with others in their areas of expertise and to exchange best practices.

Many training programs are available locally or regionally, so travel expenses can be kept to a minimum.

- *Webinars.* The numbers of Webinars and tele-seminars that offer a solid learning experience (although without the peer interaction) are increasing. They are usually inexpensive, and multiple people with similar roles in the practice can participate.
- *In-service training.* In-service training allows physicians, support staff members, or guests to provide training to the practice staff. For example, the clinical staff may meet each month to learn or refine their clinical knowledge or skills, or they may share the latest shortcuts discovered for the electronic medical record system software. The business staff may meet monthly to discuss the practice management system. Having a peer prepare and share new knowledge or skills can be a confidence builder for that employee. Physicians can also become involved in sharing their knowledge with each other and with support staff members.
- *Staff meetings.* We recommend two types of staff meetings. The first is a stand-up staff meeting that should include front- and back-office staff each week. The manager facilitates this twenty-minute session as the team literally stands in a circle to discuss, for example, customer service and physician productivity issues. The second type recommended is a monthly meeting, about an hour long, in which the support staff and physicians discuss practice performance and issues affecting the entire team. Each of these formal meetings can become an excellent forum for continuous training.

Regardless of the forum used, training topics should be identified by the manager and the POC and should be scheduled well in advance. Staff members should be paid for their attendance at these sessions, and attendance should be expected. Only with these conditions will training receive the attention it deserves in support of performance initiatives.

Leadership Development

Leadership development is another critical topic that cannot be ignored by medical practice networks. The challenges of the health care industry and the local marketplace; the increasing complexity of integrated health care; the difficulty of balancing clinical quality, service quality, physician productivity, and financial viability; and the need for "partnership led" organizations all demand the most effective leadership available. Within a hospital-owned medical practice network, that leadership must be present at three critical levels: operational governance, network management, and practice management.

In evaluating physician and administrative leaders over the years, we have used the following working definition of effective leadership:

> *Effective* is defined as providing clear direction, achieving performance targets, engaging others in accomplishing the desired results, improving organizational performance, overcoming barriers to change, motivating others to higher levels of performance, organizing work efficiently, communicating effectively, ensuring quality care and caring, and developing a culture of accountability.

More elegant definitions of leadership have been published, but this working definition has served us well.

This definition can be applied to various leadership roles from governance to frontline supervisors. For example, does the NOC establish and communicate a clear direction or performance expectation to the organization? Does accountability start with the NOC asking the network executive specific questions to determine whether or not he is implementing network-wide initiatives on time and within budget? Does the practice manager engage the POC in objective discussion about barriers to performance? Does she, in return, receive clear direction and the support to hold staff members accountable to deliver the desired result? The answers to these and similar questions yield a reliable leadership profile.

A few effective leaders seem to come by their gift naturally. The rest of us need to have an interest in and be willing to work to develop the skills necessary to consistently perform as effective leaders. Academic degrees do not guarantee leadership ability or effectiveness, nor does one's position in the organization. Having an MD or DO degree does not guarantee that the vice president of medical affairs will be effective any more than having a master's of health administration or an MBA guarantees that the chief executive officer (CEO) will be successful. Many organizations have learned this fact through experience. I have known several very effective hospital CEOs, some of whom happen to be physicians. I have met a few other CEOs who were so ineffective that I questioned how they managed to attain and retain the top seat in an organization.

Formal leadership development should be consistently pursued for those involved in operational governance and those who manage implementation, regardless of their academic background. Formally training all leaders simultaneously in certain topics has some key advantages over sending one or two away to a seminar. For example, training all leaders simultaneously in effective dialogue demonstrates the participating CEO's commitment to the principles of dialogue, provides a common vocabulary for the participants to use, and makes it safe to experiment with the principles learned (permission granted by the sponsored training). The NOC should ensure that formal training opportunities are available for its members and, where appropriate, for POC members. The network executive should make sure that formal training opportunities are made available to managers/implementers.

Less formal training and coaching opportunities are readily available through normal organizational activities. Preparing for NOC meetings places the CEO, the physician chairperson, and the network executive in monthly contact, where an experienced CEO can coach and mentor. The network executive should meet with managers on a frequent basis to provide operational feedback, training, and coaching as appropriate.

Accountability

Most organizations do a fairly good job of assigning responsibility. Many leaders adequately authorize (give permission for) their employees to act in those areas of responsibility. Relatively few leaders, however, consistently hold people accountable to deliver the desired result. Thankfully, most health care employees "feel" responsible to do well. But relatively few maintain rigorous performance measures, and even fewer actually *ask* physicians, managers, and support staff the hard questions about outcomes—even in this era of focus on quality. A culture of accountability is increasingly essential, as there is less "fat" to offset strategic, clinical, and tactical errors.

According to the authors of the best-selling book *Crucial Conversations: Tools for Talking When the Stakes Are High*:[6]

> In the *worst* companies, poor performers are first ignored and then transferred. In *good* companies, bosses eventually deal with problems. In the *best* companies, everyone holds everyone else accountable—regardless of level or position.

Members of the NOC set the accountability tone for the entire organization by holding the network executive accountable to implement approved network-wide initiatives effectively and efficiently. That accountability includes the use of a quarterly action plan, which documents those initiatives and their priority. On at least a monthly basis, the network executive reports to the NOC regarding his progress on each initiative. The same process is repeated by effective POCs, which hold their managers accountable to implement tactics contained in each practice site–specific action plan.

At a minimum, those in operational governance promote a culture that permits and expects dialogue around even the toughest issues. Members of the NOC and POCs hold each other accountable to sponsor correct operating principles by supporting implementation. Such accountability also includes line managers giving their direct reports frequent opportunities to discuss their successes, failures, challenges, barriers, and so forth. It includes questions like "If not, why not, and by when?" Performance and outcomes are rigorously measured and reported. Reasons for failure are acknowledged and documented as new learning takes place. Excuses and blame shifting are not tolerated. These factors are the essence of a culture of accountability found in successful practices.[7]

Compensation

Most hospital-owned medical practice network leaders create wage ranges for their medical practice employees that differ from the ranges found in the hospital business. We recommend that support staff wage ranges be set between the 50th and 75th percentiles for similarly situated employees in the community. This approach allows practices to potentially hire and retain a higher-quality employee. (We say "potentially" because so many other factors affect selection and retention.)

Physician compensation is an infinitely more complex matter. Medical practice success is largely a function of patient *volume* and the resulting revenue. Volume, in turn, is largely a function of physician *productivity,* and physician productivity is largely a function of the physician *compensation* approach. When employed physicians were in private practice as entrepreneurs, they were motivated by the need to meet a payroll every other week. Regardless of the income distribution approach used by the physician-owners, the support staff always got paid first. If money was left, the physicians were paid. This was essentially an "eat what you treat" model that continually motivated physicians to maintain a full schedule.

The most successful physicians were always conscious of the number of visits, surgeries, or deliveries necessary to meet their overhead expenses and the additional volume necessary to pay themselves. The most successful private practice models motivated productivity in three very important ways: First, personal and substantial risk to the physician-owners was inherent; second, the rewards or consequences of behavior (the feedback) were experienced in a timely way (every payday); third, physicians had some direct control over their personal income within a reasonable range because they could make themselves available for services (accessibility). When these same principles are applied to hospital-employed physician compensation approaches, employed physician productivity returns to private practice levels—in our experience increasing 20 percent to 30 percent or more within weeks. When these principles are ignored, employed physician productivity, as measured by work relative value units (wRVUs) or visit volume, languishes below the 50th percentile, and often below the 25th percentile, when compared with Medical Group Management Association statistics for various specialties.[8]

We often say "When you have seen one physician compensation model, you've seen one physician compensation model." While a variety of compensation approaches are available for employed physicians, those that include substantial personal risk, timely rewards, and income control tend to produce the best outcomes in terms of productivity and bottom line results—both short term and long term. Looking at common compensation approaches in light of these three critical factors is informative.

Salary

The salary approach offers physicians the most protection and security of any compensation approach. This model is best used for physicians who are new to a market and just building their practices. It is easy to define but offers little in terms of timely incentive or control over personal income.

As new practices mature, the lack of incentive can create motivational issues. Productive physicians become discouraged that they are not rewarded for building a substantial practice. Their less productive counterparts have little incentive to reach beyond their comfort levels (often only slightly above residency volumes) to build viable practices.

Bottom Line Approach

We have seen several bottom line physician compensation models that motivate productivity and practice viability. Bottom line models place physicians at risk. Rewards can be determined and distributed in a timely manner, and physicians can have substantial influence over their personal income levels. Bottom line models work because they duplicate many factors found in private practice that provide appropriate incentive. Physicians are directly motivated to see patients and motivated to code their services properly to generate revenues. Some proponents of the bottom line approach also note the potential connection to expense management.

Bottom line models, however, can pose several challenges in a hospital-owned setting, the most important of which is physicians' lack of control over several of the twelve critical revenue and expense factors as enumerated in figure 7-2. For example, many not-for-profit hospital employers require employed physicians to become an extension of the community safety net provided by emergency departments to the uninsured and underinsured populations, wreaking havoc on the practice payer mix and the resulting reimbursement. Other hospital medical practice owners turn the revenue cycle management process over to hospital central billing, with disastrous results in terms of bottom line collections.

Figure 7-2. Twelve Critical Revenue and Expense Factors

Revenue Enhancement	Expense Control
• Volume/capacity mix • Payer mix • Fees for service • Customer service • Provider productivity • Coding and documentation • Revenue cycle management • Service mix	• Physician compensation and benefits • Support staff compensation and benefits • Building occupancy • Clinical supplies

Many hospitals strip out or fail to add ancillary services to the practices they own, reducing practice revenue and physician income potential. Finally, physicians have substantial influence over only one of the four most significant expenses in a medical practice: the use of clinical supplies. The other three and most substantial expense factors—physician compensation, support staff compensation, and building occupancy—are relatively fixed in the short term, with the obvious exception of controlling support staff overtime.

Work Relative Value Unit Models

Work relative value unit models have proven to be a best practice for hospital-owned medical practices. They have several potential advantages and only a few disadvantages. For example, wRVU models focus on issues the physician can control. If the wRVU model is designed properly, it promotes substantial risk, timely reward, and significant control over personal income levels. Our consulting team has used a wRVU model for several years in a variety of settings with several specialties and have achieved positive results.

A well-designed model promotes productivity and improves procedure coding. Physicians can be payer blind in the examination room because they are paid based on services performed rather than dollars collected. As long as the charges are accurately entered into the practice management system (a local practice cashier function), the physician is paid regardless of the success or failure of the billing process.

Our recommended model includes the following factors:

Base pay = 50–70 percent of total compensation

([Prior year wRVUs × Rate per wRVU] × 0.5)/Number of pay periods

Productivity pay = 30–50 percent of total compensation and paid monthly

(Most recent three-month moving average wRVUs × Rate per wRVU) × 0.5

The wRVU model solves the payer mix issue identified in the bottom line approach. It also eliminates the risk of poor billing practices on the part of hospital central billing offices. Because many ancillary services have little or no wRVU value, the impact of stripping out ancillary services is reduced (at least as far as physician compensation is concerned), and the rate per wRVU can be set to permit a market rate of pay regardless of ancillary revenue decisions. Once physicians become accustomed to the wRVU approach, they can literally (and we encourage them to) estimate what they generated in terms of income on a daily basis.

The wRVU model does not tie the physician to the bottom line. This problem can be addressed by making practice viability a minimum performance standard. The greatest challenge for those practices using a wRVU model is establishing the right pay rate per wRVU. Balancing the need to generate a market rate of pay with the need for practice viability is the essence of that challenge. The wRVU approach must be combined with effective governance and competent management in order to address both physician compensation and practice financial viability.

Other Physician Compensation Factors

Some compensation model engineers add components in an attempt to address clinical quality, service quality, expense control, personal behavior, and other factors. In our experience, these additional components can actually detract from the desired outcome. They do so for the following reasons, each of which is discussed below:

- Complexity
- Dilution
- Measurement
- Timeliness
- Surrogate for personal accountability

Complexity

A key to the success of physician compensation models is simplicity. Ideally, physicians should be able to understand how they fared today based on their decisions today. Such immediate feedback on performance promotes continued experimentation, innovation, and achievement. Visit volumes, wRVUs, and other volume measures are ideal vehicles for providing such feedback.

Dilution

Additional components dilute the focus on productivity, which is the key driver for success because it promotes access. Assuming an adequate number of patients is available, no other factor has more to do with productivity than the compensation model. High physician productivity (above the midpoint for the specialty) is the clearest indicator that the current approach is working. Low physician productivity in the presence of adequate potential volume is the sign of a flawed compensation model. (Other factors may also negatively influence physician productivity, as illustrated in the medical practice clinical productivity evaluation presented in Appendix H.)

Measurement

Part of the challenge of other compensation model components is the difficulty of establishing reliable measures. Clinical quality is certainly challenging to define and measure. Even the simplest measures of procedural outcomes often elude detection because they are difficult to ascertain. Similarly problematic is attempting to measure the success of cognitive services, considering many patients' conditions would have improved anyway and patient compliance, or lack thereof, is often a significant variable in the equation.

Timeliness

The time between the behavior or decision and the reward is another significant challenge for many additional compensation model components. For example, patient satisfaction surveys can be reliable indicators of service quality over time, and survey questions can be directed specifically at physician interaction. Surveys are, however, expensive to randomly and continuously administer and properly interpret. Even quarterly surveys reward January behaviors in April—hardly a prescription for timely recognition.

My team and I are very interested in rigorous performance measurement for every performance driver in a medical practice or any other health care setting. Measuring clinical quality, eliminating medical errors, and identifying and implementing best practices are high priorities for every thoughtful health care professional, clinical or otherwise. Understanding service quality and optimizing the service experience for every patient and referring physician relate to another of our four critical success filters: Our commitment to quality in both areas is unquestionable. Quality, however, is not good fodder for an effective physician compensation model because such measures fail to place the physician at substantial risk and fail to support timely rewards.

Surrogate for Personal Accountability

Should we reward a licensed professional for "good citizenship" or for providing quality care? We do not reward support staff for being "nice." Such behavior is expected and is the minimum standard for continued employment. If a receptionist offends multiple patients, the practice terminates its relationship with that employee. Even more than minimum standards is expected of licensed professionals—at least those we want to have as business partners.

On one occasion, we became aware that one of our clients' employed physicians was months behind on charting. Sticky notes containing cryptic comments had been applied to hundreds of charts as documentation reminders. The physician was a wonderful doctor with a great bedside manner and a huge patient following. All evidence indicated that he was clinically competent, as well. However, his practice partners complained about having to see his patients without clear progress notes. His staff complained about the constant search for incomplete charts that were found in his office or in the trunk of his car. Patients were obviously at increasing risk. Coding could not be easily verified, even though bills were sent out based on fee tickets completed at the time of service. Worst of all, this pattern had been tolerated for years.

With the encouragement of the risk management office, the help of a dedicated office manager and staff, and the support of physician partners, current patient scheduling was placed on hold so the physician could catch up on his charting. Formal notice, a timeline for completion, and consequences for failure to perform were provided. Unfortunately, the physician did not adequately comply with the terms of the notice, even when additional time was provided. His contract was terminated. While the foregoing represents an extreme case, such performance issues are not unheard of among employed physicians—some of whom could not succeed in a private practice setting if exhibiting these behaviors.

The safety net of hospital employment under the wrong compensation approach and without accountability (including consequences for unprofessional behavior) permits some situations to last for years and requires far more attention, in terms of management resources, than they deserve. Personal accountability for appropriate behavior is a minimum standard for remaining part of the team. Rewarding minimum standard behavior as part of a compensation model is unnecessary and dilutes the more important, productive behaviors that influence success.

Mid-level Provider Compensation

Mid-level practitioners in a traditional practice setting provide medical services and generate wRVUs. Where mid-level providers are allowed to develop their own patient following, they should also participate in a productivity-based compensation approach similar to that of employed physicians, at a rate per wRVU that is commensurate with their specialty and fair-market compensation. In practices where mid-level providers are used as physician extenders and not allowed to develop their own patient populations, a productivity model may not work effectively.

For those practices transitioning from a salary model to a productivity model, we recommend that the physicians transition first, as their productivity will improve. This improvement will expand the physicians' access to their patients, many of whom prefer to see a physician over a mid-level provider. Once the volume has shifted and settled, mid-level providers can successfully transition to a productivity approach. We usually recommend a six-month lag between the physicians shifting and the mid-level providers participating in the model. This lag allows time for overall practice volume to grow and gives mid-level providers an opportunity to expand their practices.

Employee Benefits

Without question, most of our client hospitals and health systems have elected to offer their substantial employee benefit packages to all employees. This gesture is often supported by discussions of internal equity and other ethical considerations. It can also be supported by ease of administration. Unfortunately, hospital-level benefits are not financially sustainable as part of a medical practice cost structure and often guarantee financial operating losses in the owned practices. This approach also places additional pressure on private practices in the community to increase benefits in order to retain their employees, driving up their operating costs as small employers.

We encourage hospital and health system clients to reconsider this approach. As large entities, they can still offer modified (lesser) employee benefit packages that are very competitive with local market employers (including independent physicians) and much more sustainable in a medical practice setting. Similar to offering unique wage ranges for support staff in their owned medical practices, hospitals should offer support staff benefits that are relevant to community medical practices and other similar employers, thereby maintaining community equity and reducing artificial benefit inflation (resetting the market norm by imposing an unsustainable standard on others).

Physician Employment Contract Highlights

Some hospital executives have been forced through experience to recognize the challenges associated with establishing separate deals with various employed physicians. Negotiating and renegotiating varied employment contracts require huge amounts of energy for management and the physicians immediately involved. The perception of "better deals" offered to peers becomes a significant distraction for employed physicians (e.g., "My partner pulled up in a new Mercedes after renegotiating his contract with the hospital CEO, who is his golfing buddy."). A standard contract for all employed physicians eliminates both of these issues and is a best practice.

Some nuanced adjustments for invasive versus cognitive specialties will be necessary. For example, given the nature of family practice, a five-mile radius noncompete clause is usually adequate to protect the practice and the hospital. A surgery practice may need a fifteen-mile radius to achieve the same level of market share protection.

When we negotiate an employment contract with a new physician, we start with a term sheet, as discussed in chapter 5, that highlights the deal in lay terms. Term sheets are not as intimidating as employment contracts and generally include relevant topics such as those illustrated as Appendix D.

Once the term sheet has been discussed and its content agreed upon, the practice will be prepared to present and explain the formal employment contract document containing the more challenging and potentially intimidating legal language.

Summary

I have heard managers complain that if it were not for people and computers, their lives would be perfect. I suspect that most managers have days when they share such sentiments.

At the same time, no experience is more rewarding in the workplace than working with a group of people who gel and become a true team. The power, synergy, innovation, and commitment emanating from such a team are adequate to surmount any barriers to providing top-quality care in a caring environment. The foundation of that team is a group of A players who understand and do their work under the direction of a skilled leader. Those A players include physicians, managers, and support staff members who not only feel accountable but are held accountable for their behavior and outcomes.

Fielding a team of A players certainly involves appropriate selection. Perhaps even more important to development is training, motivation, and a culture of accountability. Because the medical practice business is heavily dependent on the physician's skill and motivation, practice viability also involves the implementation of a physician compensation model that motivates high levels of productivity, which elevate expectations for the entire practice.

References

1. M. Halley and M. Ferry, *The Medical Practice Start-Up Guide,* 69–93 (Phoenix, MD: Greenbranch, 2008).
2. P. Drucker, *Peter Drucker on the Profession of Management,* 122 (Boston: Harvard Business School Publishing, 1998).
3. J. Carlzon, *Moments of Truth: New Strategies for Today's Customer-Driven Economy* (New York: Harper and Row, 1987).
4. F. Herzberg, "One More Time: How Do You Motivate Employees?" *Harvard Business Review* September/October (1987): 5–6.
5. S. Certo, *Supervision: Quality, Diversity, and Technology,* 547–548 (Chicago: McGraw-Hill, 1997).
6. Kerry Patterson, Joseph Grenny, Ron McMillan, and Al Switzler, *Crucial Conversations: Tools for Talking When the Stakes Are High,* 11 (New York: McGraw-Hill, 2002).
7. M. Halley, "A Culture of Accountability: What Distinguishes an Exceptional Medical Group." *Group Practice Journal* 54, no. 3 (2005): 11–14.
8. Medical Group Management Association, *Physician Compensation and Production Survey* (Englewood, CO: Medical Group Management Association, 2009).

CHAPTER 8

Practice and Network Operations

Achieving success in a hospital-owned medical practice network requires attention to initiatives, such as a more effective physician compensation model or a new practice management system, that can improve (sometimes dramatically) the performance of the entire physician network. These network-wide initiatives alone, however, will not drive the network to financial viability. Medical practice networks ultimately achieve performance targets one practice, or even one physician, at a time.

Practice operations councils (POCs) and their practice managers must focus on twelve critical success factors *within each practice* to attain and maintain operational and financial viability. Those factors were introduced in chapter 7 (figure 7-2) and are further defined in the paragraphs that follow.

Critical Success Factors

As we recall, the success of a practice is largely a function of revenue, which is largely a function of volume, which is largely a function of physician productivity, which is largely a function of the physician compensation arrangement. However, physician productivity is only one of eight factors affecting the revenue side of the income statement. Many of these factors, introduced in chapter 2 and listed below, influence or are influenced by practice and network operations:

- Volume/capacity mix
- Payer mix
- Fees for service
- Customer service
- Physician productivity
- Coding and documentation
- Revenue cycle management
- Service mix

The following four critical expense factors constitute nearly 85 percent of a traditional medical practice cost structure:

- Physician compensation and benefits
- Support staff compensation and benefits
- Building occupancy
- Clinical supplies

Once again, these four expense factors are all influenced by network and practice operations. Regardless of ownership, medical practice success is dependent on success in *each* revenue and expense area.

Network Operations Management

Network operations management is the implementation process for the network operations council (NOC). It includes those issues, decisions, and policies that cross practice boundaries, affecting more than one cost center, and are dealt with by the NOC and network executive. Collectively, they are known as *network-wide initiatives.*

It is critical for NOCs and executives to realize that while network-wide initiatives can support performance improvement, the only way to ultimately achieve clinical excellence, outstanding service quality, high productivity, and financial viability is on a practice-by-practice—or even physician-by-physician—basis. For this reason, NOCs must do all they can to push relevant decisions and accountability for those decisions to the practice level.

Still, in network settings, it is logical that decisions about physician capacity, payer mix strategy, fees, revenue cycle management, the physician compensation model, staff wage ranges, employee benefits, group purchasing, practice management systems, and electronic medical record (EMR) systems, among others, end up being defined as network-wide initiatives. While several network-wide topics are addressed in other chapters, a few of them are particularly relevant to this operations management chapter and are discussed below.

Volume/Capacity Mix

Matching physician (and mid-level provider) capacity to current and potential patient volume is certainly a marketing and practice development issue. It is also a network operations issue, especially critical in markets that are saturated with the specialty in question and in those with significant need but without an adequate population to fill an additional physician practice.

Saturated markets become a zero sum game, whereby a physician must steal every new patient from another physician in the same geographic area. Alternatively, a distant rural community with a population of 2,500 needs and deserves a physician or another provider, but capturing that entire population will not fill a productive practice. A growing practice that has outstripped the capacity of the existing physicians and other providers is another common network development challenge. Each of these and similar scenarios are usually best addressed or reconciled at the network operations level.

The decision to add physician capacity to a particular practice or neighborhood in support of an integrated strategy will be addressed at the NOC. *Which* physician to add to a small group practice should be the decision of the relevant POC, which will share its practice with the new physician. The decision to place a new physician or another provider in a new practice in a new neighborhood in support of an integrated strategy will be addressed at the NOC, with the hospital chief executive officer signing the employment contract and supporting the attendant start-up salary and operating costs with capital.

Fees for Service

Fees for the services provided are a marketing issue, a revenue cycle issue, a financial issue, and sometimes a legal/regulatory structural issue (e.g., provider-based reimbursement). Generally, however, fees are established at the network level as a network operations matter. They are usually common to all practices and specialties in the network and are based on analysis of reimbursement experience across the network. Multispecialty networks face additional complexity in establishing fees and should frequently audit the explanation-of-benefits information that accompanies reimbursement to ensure that payers are meeting their contractual obligations (contract management) and that fees are appropriate for the services provided. Fees should be reviewed annually, at a minimum.

Payer Mix

Establishing the appropriate payer mix is a mission issue, an ethical issue, a potential legal/regulatory issue, a strategy issue, and a marketing and practice development issue. Whether a hospital is a for-profit or a not-for-profit facility, care of the uninsured and underinsured is a significant matter that continues to receive local, regional, and national attention. From a purely selfish financial perspective, hospitals that fail to care for those who are in need often end up addressing subsequent tragedies, at a much higher cost, in their emergency rooms. For some patients, the costs of these lifesaving services are high enough to bankrupt those unfortunate enough to require them, who are either uninsured or whose health insurance places limits on reimbursement.

At the same time, hospitals and medical practices that do not manage their payer mix may soon find themselves unable to meet payroll. Without setting limits, a new primary care physician will become inundated with the uninsured and underinsured members of the community presenting as patients. Specialty physicians with referrals coming only from primary care physicians in poorer neighborhoods will not be able to offer competitive compensation to new partners and will soon burn out. Hospitals that draw patients only from those same economically challenged neighborhoods will have a difficult time amassing the capital necessary to remain viable in terms of technology, facilities, or human capital.

Payer mix issues cannot be legislated or regulated away or solved by a generous mission statement. They cannot be resolved by imposing guilt on investors or the threat of taxation on not-for-profit sponsors. Nor can payers be expected to take on inordinate risk without increasing premiums for those who can pay if they are to remain viable and continue to insure against risk. While I do not pretend to have an answer for this complex problem, and I am not so bold as to offer counsel on appropriate levels of profit or provider compensation (how much is enough?), I have seen a number of efforts that provide partial relief to the current situation while keeping the providers viable to fight another day. A few of these ideas follow:

- We have seen community hospitals cooperate to ensure the success of Federally Qualified Health Centers that receive reimbursement in excess of private practices for Medicaid patients.
- We have seen hospitals designate certain practices in their networks as mission practices, equipped and staffed with the same quality equipment and professional-level staff as non-mission locations.
- We have seen hospital-owned practices implement charity care policies that provide assistance for those who demonstrate that they are truly needy and do not have the ability to pay all or a portion of their medical fees.
- We have seen hospitals successfully implement Provider-Based Status or Rural Health Clinic strategies to supplement their reimbursement for services to the underserved.
- We have seen practices cooperate with pharmaceutical companies to provide medication to their needy patients.
- We have seen physicians and other providers contribute a portion of their time to work in free clinics, including employed physicians whose employers support their efforts.
- We have seen practices accept a fair portion of the uninsured and underinsured and then refer additional new patients to mission locations supported by their networks.
- We have seen specialty physicians employed by hospitals and paid based on work relative value units take a disproportionate share of Medicaid and uninsured patients to take the pressure off of independent specialists who still must meet a payroll, particularly in areas where a large portion of the population is uninsured or underinsured.

We recommend that hospital-owned medical practice networks strive to become and remain financially viable. To accomplish this objective, most of their practices must become and remain financially viable. They cannot do so without setting limits on certain payers—just like private practices. At the same time, the network can offer every patient the option to visit the practice(s) and see physicians and mid-level providers designated to serve the underserved, uninsured, and underinsured. The result is good business, good ethics, and quality care.

Human Resource Issues

A variety of human resource issues are related to network operations policies and decisions and are implemented network-wide as network operations initiatives. These areas include common physician employment contracts, a common provider compensation model, a common employee benefits package, a common wage scale for support staff, and common human resource policies. Commonality in these areas helps ensure compliance with labor laws and helps prevent any "special deals" that can become prevalent in less well organized networks, creating discord and mistrust.

Group Purchasing

Group purchasing has always been a significant cost containment strategy for hospitals and health systems. Quite naturally, then, it makes its way into the medical practices owned and operated by those hospitals—sometimes as a benefit, but often as a source of frustration. For most physician specialties, expendable clinical supplies and pharmaceuticals are the fourth largest cost category but only account for 3 percent to 6 percent of net patient revenue. (One notable exception is oncology, depending on the accounting for drugs.) Office supplies usually account for 1 percent or 2 percent of the cost structure. Still, some practices benefit from joining large group purchasing arrangements. Other private practices find that their supply costs increase after they are acquired by hospitals and forced into group purchasing arrangements. Still others find that service levels decline and they must increase inventories to account for the poorer service.

Some years ago, I tried to order one bottle of Betadine solution for a new solo internal medicine (IM) practice. I called the hospital purchasing department (as instructed) and was told that I would need to order a case of Betadine because the department would distribute only cases to the hospital floors. After explaining, in vain, that a case of Betadine could not be used in ten years in a solo IM practice, I violated policy and bought a bottle from the local pharmacy. We encourage our clients to use the hospital's group purchasing process where that participation makes sense, remembering that it is a "hospital" group purchasing process.

Practice Operations Management

Practice operations management is the implementation process for POCs. It deals with practice- or site-specific factors and with the implementation of network-wide initiatives at the practice level. Such issues as payer mix management;

service quality; point-of-service collections; physician productivity; coding and documentation; service mix; hiring, training, and scheduling support staff; ordering supplies; and inventory control should dominate the agenda for POCs and practice managers. The following paragraphs address best practices in some of the most significant practice operations topics.

Critical Success Filters

While all four critical success filters—clinical quality, service quality, physician productivity, and operational and financial viability—should affect strategies, policies, procedures, designs, and decisions at every level of the medical practice network, success or failure for all four filters is largely a function of local practice operations. Implementation of clinical quality initiatives must occur at the practice level. The service quality "rubber meets the road" at the appointment desk, in the reception area, in the examination room, and at the cashier's station. Physician and mid-level productivity is largely influenced by what happens in the "productivity zone," which includes the examination rooms, the nurse's station, and the doctor's work station. And the first three filters affect the financial viability of the practice operation, regardless of practice ownership. Optimizing literally every aspect of practice operations includes consideration of these four filters.

Highest and Best-Use Staffing

The myriad roles in a medical practice can be divided into two categories. Primary roles are those that have the most significant impact on the overall service experience of the medical practice customers (patients and referring physicians). Those roles are the physician, the mid-level provider, the clinical assistant, and the receptionist. All other jobs and roles are secondary roles and assist or support the primary roles in ensuring a top-quality experience for every customer, every time. Those in secondary roles often see the patients or occasionally interact with referring physicians, but the primary roles have the most significant impact.

The key to the success of highest and best-use staffing[1] is to ensure that the primary roles are not encumbered with duties that do not relate to their area of responsibility. The physician does what only a physician can do and delegates everything else. The clinical assistant does what only the clinical assistant can do and delegates everything else. The receptionist focuses on receiving patients and is unencumbered by anything that does not support the greeting and an efficient process for checking patients into the practice.

THE RECEPTIONIST

A highest and best-use receptionist, for example, greets each patient warmly, efficiently gathers or verifies the patient's personal information, collects the co-payment, and makes sure the patient is comfortably seated in the reception room. Some receptionists think their responsibilities end once the patient is seated and waiting for the clinical assistant to call. Highest and best-use receptionists, however, are like lifeguards, watching every bobbing head in the reception area until the clinical assistant calls the patient back to the examination room.

Such receptionists know what time each patient checked into the office and how long he or she has been waiting. They are quick to apologize for any inordinate delay (usually more than fifteen minutes) and are scripted to express the physician's concern about the patient's time. They may even ask if the patient can continue to wait. In doing so, they let the customer know that he or she has not been forgotten—a much appreciated gesture.

Such receptionists cannot be bothered with numerous phone calls or excessive data entry duties. Everything they do must be focused on receiving and monitoring the customers until they are handed off to the clinical assistant.

THE CLINICAL ASSISTANT

The highest and best-use clinical assistant has two critical responsibilities: to help ensure that the patient receives high-quality care in a caring environment and to drive physician productivity. The term *drive* is used purposely. While physicians are in the examination room, they are totally engaged (at least we hope) in the physical examination, diagnosis, and treatment planning for an individual patient. As a patient, I want my physician totally absorbed with me and my issue(s), not watching the clock. Unfortunately, an office visit can quickly deteriorate into a social call involving that most expensive practice resource. Many physicians have a difficult time extracting themselves from social calls without outside help.

A highest and best-use clinical assistant knows how long the patient's chief complaint should take and politely taps on the door once that time limit is reached. When invited, the assistant opens the door and lets the physician know the he is needed "in exam room 2." Assuming all is well, the physician can excuse himself, and that "nice nurse" who took my blood pressure is back to continue the conversation while closing down the visit and accompanying me to the cashier's station. If, on the other hand, the clinical assistant knocks on the door and the physician holds up his index finger as she enters, she knows that he has indeed discovered something unanticipated and immediately offers to help.

If the clinical assistant is appropriately monitoring those three examination rooms (in a cognitive practice, for example), the physician can easily see one, two, or even more additional patients in a day. Unfortunately, clinical assistants are not always focused on driving physician productivity. They may be on the telephone with a hospital department trying to schedule a diagnostic test or working with an insurance company on a referral. They may be hunting for a chart, scanning the physician's mail, and completing referral tracking information.

Highest and best-use staffing involves removing from that clinical assistant role every task that does not promote quality patient care and caring and does not drive physician productivity. Implementing highest and best-use staffing, then, may mean the practice needs to hire another medical assistant or nurse to handle those "other duties as assigned." Some of our hospital clients raise their eyebrows when we suggest hiring more staff for a clinic that is already losing money. However, if productivity is the problem, adding that \$12 to \$22–an-hour clinical assistant to enhance the productivity of the very expensive physician resource is hard to argue with.

THE PHYSICIAN

As mentioned, highest and best-use physicians do what only physicians can do. They delegate everything else to a clinical assistant who can take the additional workload because she has been able to delegate some of her extraneous responsibilities to an extra clinical assistant or other secondary role. Ideally, the clutter of extraneous activities can be removed from the productivity zone. Removing both *physical clutter* and *role clutter* helps ensure the productivity of a properly focused work team.

Peter Anderson, MD, a family physician practicing in Roanoke, Virginia, has taken the concept of highest and best-use staffing to heart. While his work style will not fit every preference, the concepts are illustrative. He works in several examination rooms with two full-time clinical assistants seeing forty to forty-five patients a day with demonstrably high levels of clinical quality, patient satisfaction, nurse satisfaction, physician satisfaction, physician income, and financial viability.

Years ago, Dr. Anderson realized that the typical ambulatory patient visit includes four components: (1) data gathering and communication of data, (2) analysis of the data and the physical examination, (3) decision making and treatment plan development, and (4) implementation of the plan and patient education. He also realized that a competent nurse should be able to accomplish steps 1 and 4, as they provide similar services in the more complex hospital setting.

Using a set of protocols developed by Dr. Anderson, a nurse invites a patient from the reception area to an examination room and, based on the reported chief complaint, runs through the associated protocol questions. When Dr. Anderson enters the examination room, the nurse remains in the room and reports, in the presence of the patient, what she has learned during the data-gathering phase. Dr. Anderson asks clarifying questions as needed, and the patient has the opportunity to enhance the information reported. The physician then conducts the physical examination and diagnoses the patient. While doing so, he shares with the nurse what he wants placed in the chart (now an EMR).

Dr. Anderson decides on a treatment plan and shares that plan with the patient and the nurse; the nurse then documents it in the EMR. Dr. Anderson leaves the examination room, allowing the nurse to provide additional instruction, offer relevant patient education materials, and close the visit by accompanying the patient to the cashier station. In the meantime, Dr. Anderson is in the next examination room with the second nurse, who has the next patient prepared. Again, while this approach may not match a particular physician's practice style or specialty, it is an illustration of highest and best-use staffing.[2]

In our experience, the most productive cognitive specialties have *higher* numbers of support staff but a *lower* labor ratio (support staff costs divided by net patient revenue). These practices have discovered that higher levels of support staff can, if roles are properly defined, leverage the physician by enhancing her productivity and generating revenue far in excess of the additional labor costs.

Work Flow and Job Design

A number of factors affect work flow in a particular medical practice setting. These factors include, but are not limited to:

- Objectives for quality care and caring
- The physician specialty
- Referral and patient volume
- The size of the practice (e.g., number of physicians)
- The size and design of the physical plant
- The clinical and business equipment available to support human resources
- The capabilities and experience of the physician(s) (e.g., interest in performing procedures in the practice setting)
- The capabilities and experience of the support staff (e.g., registered nurses versus certified medical assistants)
- The patient profile (e.g., geriatric and pediatric patients, who each present unique challenges)
- The physician's practice style (e.g., some physicians who are slower and more methodical than others)
- The physician's personal productivity and motivation
- The appointment scheduling method
- The ancillary services available in the practice
- Legal/contractual and regulatory requirements
- The capabilities of practice software (e.g., the practice management and EMR systems)
- Management requirements
- Hours of operation

PROCESS IMPROVEMENT

Medical practices develop, formally or by default, methods or processes (a series of steps) to manage the work flow. Again, formally or otherwise, those processes or steps become part of "jobs" as they are delegated to various individuals within the practice. That is, they become part of roles (ideally documented in job descriptions) for receptionists, appointment clerks, medical records clerks, clinical assistants, even physicians and other providers.

Unfortunately, work flow factors are far from static. They change over time—sometimes rapidly. Consequently, processes that were once logical evolve as incumbents implement process "fixes" in response to continuous changes in their work flows. Again, over time, processes can become bogged down by the weight of these expediencies, reducing both effectiveness and efficiency. As effectiveness and efficiency decline, the ability to provide quality care and caring are negatively affected, regardless of ability, commitment, and motivation levels.

Newer practices with few referring physicians and low patient volumes may perform adequately using sloppy methods, but the busier they become, the more efficient and effective their processes must become in order to survive. Established practices must vigilantly monitor key processes to ensure that they are still meeting their intended purpose (still effective) with a reasonable expenditure of resources (still efficient). Failure to manage processes in response to changes in one or more of the above-mentioned factors ensures that work flow will bog down over time. A simple case in point may illustrate the concept.

Not long ago my wife encouraged me to see the dermatologist she uses. As in most communities, her dermatologist had a two-month wait for new patients, so I lined up. On the appointed day, I arrived about fifteen minutes early to complete the new-patient paperwork. I walked up to the reception desk with my insurance card and driver's license in hand. I was handed a clipboard full of paperwork for the practice.

The paperwork was most interesting. In the space of about ten minutes, I had to write and rewrite my name five times—not because I couldn't get it right, but because several different documents required it. I had to write my social security number three times and my insurance group number at least twice. While redundancy for me is a frustration, redundancy for the doctor's support staff is costly. As I examined the forms, I saw that much of the redundancy could be eliminated with a cover sheet and staple, redesigned multipurpose sheets, prenumbered attachments, carbonless paper, or a variety of other techniques.

This experience reminded me of a quote I memorized in graduate school. Although I cannot find the source, I recall that it goes like this: "Every organization is a coral reef of policies and procedures established to achieve some long-forgotten objective." The term *coral reef* implies rigid structures built on previous foundations. I suspect that the dermatology practice new-patient packet, over time, evolved to meet new demands, prevent errors, incorporate somebody's great idea, and so forth. By the time I received it, it had become the official method, or "the way we do things around here."

WORK FLOW ANALYSIS

Work flow, of course, is a local phenomenon and must be identified and improved site by site within a medical practice network. Practice operations councils and their practice managers must be involved in developing or revising work processes in response to changes in work flow factors that occur in or are imposed on the practice setting.

Work flow analysis can be as simple as listing the steps in the process. For example, consider the process of adding a new patient to a specialty practice. The following steps may apply:

1. Physician referral
2. Appointment call
3. Preliminary patient information gathered
4. Referring physician profile checked
5. Appointment scheduled
6. New-patient packet sent
7. Preauthorization, as required
8. Referring physician called according to profile
9. Progress note to tickler file, as needed
10. Patient reminder call
11. Patient arrival and greeting
12. New-patient information reviewed and verified
13. Co-payment collected, as required
14. Patient comfortably seated
15. Patient kept informed
16. Patient greeted by nurse

At least sixteen steps occur before the specialty physician meets the patient for the first time. These are the "moments of truth," discussed in chapter 6. Managing these moments of truth properly sets the tone for the patient's experience in the specialty practice, which will likely be communicated to the referring physician. So the first process improvement focus is to define a successful outcome for each moment or step. Remember, some of these steps will be subdivided into tasks that must be accomplished in order to ensure that the step is successful.

A properly functioning process has the following characteristics:

- The desired outcome and performance expectations for the process and each individual step and task are clearly defined. For example, the referring physician telephone line is answered by a competent human being within three rings.

- Each task contributes to the defined outcome by accomplishing its intended purpose (effectiveness) without damaging clinical quality, service quality, or physician productivity.
- Each task accomplishes its intended purpose by using the proper resources (efficiency) while maintaining clinical quality, service quality, and provider productivity. For example, receptionists are not practicing medicine, and doctors are not using the fax machine.
- Each task contributes to (or does not detract from) the efficiency and effectiveness of subsequent tasks.
- Tasks are grouped with like tasks into roles and jobs. For example, tasks that include numerous interruptions and scripted responses (e.g., answering the telephone) are not mixed with tasks that require creative thought and concentration (e.g., completing a performance evaluation).

In fact, testing processes by asking these and similar questions is a great way to assess the effectiveness of the process. Tasks that efficiently and effectively accomplish their intended purpose and contribute to the required performance remain part of the process. Those that do not are eliminated (preferable), revised, or replaced. The revised tasks are then assigned to jobs.

Recognizing That Size Matters

Practice size and volume do make a difference in job design. Obviously, in solo practices, with limited staff and volumes, each employee must become a "jack of all trades," able to step into a variety of roles and tasks on a daily basis. However, in larger practices with high patient volumes and multiple staff, success requires increased job specialization. Otherwise, too many jacks of all trades end up looking like the "Keystone Kops," constantly tripping over each other despite their good intentions.

For example, in small practices, the receptionist answers the telephone, sets appointments, pulls the medical chart, greets patients, verifies insurance and demographics, collects co-payments, attaches the fee ticket, enters charges, collects patient-due balances, and so forth. In larger practices, these responsibilities are divided among multiple front-office staff members who carry titles like receptionist, cashier, medical records clerk, appointments clerk, and so forth. These staff, who are specialists in their own right, can cross train to support each other, but each still has his or her specific set of tasks (or job).

Staffing to Demand

Scheduling the most important human resources is an operational function. Staffing to demand starts with scheduling the most expensive physician resources. As mentioned earlier, matching physician and other provider capacity to current and potential volume is an operations function that will likely require input from the network level and attentive management by each POC.

Once roles/jobs have been assigned to individual employees, management must schedule support staff in appropriate numbers to meet the needs, wants, and priorities of patients and their referring physicians. The numbers and types of support staff scheduled must also promote the productivity of the practice and its physicians. Failure to adequately staff to meet demand creates frustration for patients, referring physicians, practice physicians, and support staff. Understaffing also increases payroll costs, especially if it results in overtime. Overstaffing is costly as well, often resulting in lower productivity per employee as limited work expands to fill the time allotted.

Proper staffing starts with anticipated demand, usually based on the schedule of physicians and other providers. We encourage POCs to insist that physicians maintain a stable appointment schedule to provide access for patients and to facilitate staffing to demand.

Changing the appointment schedule frequently or on a whim violates at least two of the four critical success filters: service quality and physician productivity. We encourage POCs and practice managers to set the expectation that support staffing will be adjusted according to demand. For example, if a physician is not present, his or her clinical assistant usually should not be present. Overtime should be strictly avoided except for unusual and infrequent circumstances. As POCs and managers become more sophisticated in this approach, they will carefully watch the labor cost ratio (labor costs/net patient revenue) to make sure it remains within the appropriate range. Staffing objectives will likely be included in most site-specific action plans.

Payer Mix

The implementation of payer mix strategy or policy is a practice operations matter, as it is heavily dependent on the appointment clerk. The availability of appointment slots for new patients the practice can accept and properly referring new patients whom it cannot accept to alternative locations (e.g., a Federally Qualified Health Center, a designated mission-based practice) occurs largely at the appointment work station. Appointment clerks should be well trained and scripted to provide support to every person calling the practice, regardless of their insurance coverage or ability to pay. According to network-wide policies, those who call are directed to the appropriate locations.

Customer Service

Every aspect of practice operations affects customer service. All operational policies, procedures, and tasks must support effective and efficient customer service if the practice is to meet the needs, wants, and priorities of referring physicians and their patients.

While customer-focused policies and procedures and proper job design are critical to service quality, they are not enough to ensure consistent implementation. Customer service must become an ingrained part of each practice culture, led by the POC and its individual physician members. The "caring" part of high-quality care and caring has to be "the way we do things." The topic is found in one form or another on every stand-up staff meeting agenda, every all-staff meeting agenda, and every POC agenda.

Service improvement is a continuous process rather than an event. While patient satisfaction surveys and new patient ratios are indicators of success or failure in this arena, it is the daily interaction with patients that provides real-time feedback. Asking "How was your visit today?" is more than just a common courtesy. It is an inquiry meant to gather information and provide feedback *to people and on processes.*

Physician Productivity

As reimbursement continues to decline, the productivity of physicians, mid-level providers, and staff becomes increasingly critical to the continued success of medical practices. The term *productivity* sometimes elicits thoughts of assembly lines, patient mills, robotic providers, and cattle prods, which are not conducive to the practice of medicine. Experience has demonstrated, however, that physicians and their support staff can be both caring and productive, yielding a great experience for patients and their referring physicians.

Productivity is a function of physician and clinic setting factors. Appendix H is a medical practice clinical productivity evaluation that illustrates the questions that POCs and practice managers can ask to spur discussions about improving productivity in the productivity zone. This self-evaluation should be reviewed quarterly, for each physician, to ensure that productivity remains a top priority.

Coding and Documentation

For years, coding experts have been telling our clients that physicians tend to under-code and under-document for billing purposes relative to the level of care actually provided. While I cannot cite any studies to confirm this assertion, we see improvement in coding, documentation, and reimbursement almost every time we provide effective coding training to physicians.

Physicians should do their own procedure and diagnosis coding, particularly for the most common office visits and procedures. They should also understand how to properly code and document for billing purposes. Given the constant changes in coding requirements for payers, physicians and support staff should receive annual training in the latest coding updates.

We recommend that professional coders be hired to supplement that annual training throughout the year by conducting quarterly coding and documentation audits for every provider, followed by a review of findings and recommendations with each physician. Professional coders can also serve as help desk resources to research unique or uncommon situations. Under proper circumstances, we usually find that one professional coding resource can support as many as twenty-five physicians and other providers. The proper circumstances include readily available histograms to compare coding across each specialty within the network and with external benchmarks, and tools to facilitate documentation review.

Revenue Cycle Management

Effective revenue cycle management is such a common challenge for hospital-owned medical practice networks that we have dedicated a short chapter to discussion of this critical topic. (See chapter 9.)

Service Mix

As we recall from earlier chapters, service mix involves the scope of services offered in each network practice and the way access to those services is provided. From a marketing perspective, the practice provides the services that Mrs. Smith and her referring physician expect to find in its offices according to the community standard of care, including laboratory services, radiology services, screening procedures, and so forth. From an operations perspective, the practice offers those services that can meet all four critical success filters, including at least break-even financial performance. It offers those services in the place where the customer prefers them—usually in a convenient, one-stop shop.

Adding procedures and ancillary services to a medical practice does create a new dynamic that must be considered carefully in the work flow. The following issues might affect the decision to provide the service:

- Where will the service be provided? Will it be provided in the examination room, making that room unavailable for a period of time? Will a special procedure room be dedicated to service delivery?
- Will unique equipment be required? Will that equipment be mobile or fixed?
- Will special training be required for the physician and the support staff? Will special certification be needed for the providers or support staff? Will the service need to be accredited to demonstrate clinical quality in providing the service?

- What type of setup is required before the procedure, and what cleanup will be required afterward? Will facility changes be necessary to achieve effective and efficient cleanup?
- When will the service be provided? Will it be available during normal business hours (e.g., laboratory, radiology, laceration repair)? Will special times or days be required (e.g., endoscopy screening, mobile mammography, bone densitometry)?
- How will the service fit into the normal flow of patients throughout our office? Will it create additional wait time? What impact will it have on the productivity zone?
- What is the opportunity cost of providing the service? In other words, will the service more than offset the value of seeing additional patients rather than providing the service?
- Will reimbursement be adequate to cover the *total cost* of the service and contribute to our financial viability?

This list of questions should not become an excuse for failing to offer additional ancillary services. As a best practice, the bias should be to offer a more comprehensive scope of services to address patient and referring physician expectations while still meeting all four critical success filters.

Accountability

We have touched on accountability several times. Once again, it is in practice operations where accountability is most keenly felt—or missed. The practices that operate most effectively and efficiently are those in which the physicians hold each other accountable to "play by the rules." If even one physician is allowed to ignore POC policies or agreements, the entire operation is at risk. "Not my nurse!" is never heard in properly functioning offices, for example.

Special allowances are the death knell for efficient and effective practice operations. If the physicians are united in their sponsorship of policies based on correct operating principles, the practice manager can hold support staff accountable, as well. Even one allowance contrary to policy undercuts the credibility of the manager and the POC.

Every incumbent in every role within the medical practice should establish performance improvement objectives. Certainly, external standards such as accreditation requirements or benchmark statistics can form the basis of these objectives, but those should typically be viewed as minimum standards rather than performance targets. Internal performance targets that are *understood by* and *established with* incumbents, and continuous performance improvement should be the cultural norm for a successful practice.

Continuously setting and achieving targets, overcoming barriers, and celebrating successes create a different kind of team, one in which the status quo is not good enough. Whether the performance improvement topic is point-of-service collections, patient wait times, updating the immunization records, exceeding HEDIS (National Committee for Quality Assurance's Healthcare Effectiveness Data and Information Set) measures, "wowing" the patient, or responding to a referring physician, anything we understand, measure, and commit to improve, will improve. When the POC and the practice manager decide to create a high-performance team, little can impede their achievement, and high-performance teams welcome performance measures as evidence of their achievement. Low-performing individuals and teams, on the other hand, spend more time questioning the data and justifying their poor performance.

Summary

Hospital-owned medical practice networks break even and remain financially viable one practice, even one physician, at a time. Despite all the great network-wide initiatives that must and will be implemented in support of network practices, the path to viability is effective and efficient individual practice operations.

In successful practices, POCs will rigorously monitor and succeed in all eight revenue factors. They will monitor and control all four expense factors. Work flow design and division of tasks will be based on achieving high clinical quality as defined by the practice's physicians, high service quality as defined by the patients and their referring physicians, and high physician productivity. POCs and practice managers will realize that change is constantly occurring and key processes must be monitored to ensure that they remain effective and efficient. Importantly, an accountability culture will ensure the presence of A players and their continual focus on achieving the desired result.

References

1. M. Halley and M. Ferry, *The Medical Practice Start-Up Guide,* 72–74 (Phoenix, MD: Greenbranch, 2008).
2. P. Anderson and M. Halley, "A New Approach to Making Your Doctor-Nurse Team More Productive," *Family Practice Management* July/August (2008): 35–40.

CHAPTER 9

Revenue Cycle Management

In the mid-1990s, on a summer afternoon in Chicago, several of our client executives and our consulting team were gathered for our annual management retreat. The afternoon session was dedicated to addressing the pervasive revenue cycle management challenge encountered in hospital-owned medical practices. The stories shared by the executives were consistent: Hospitals that acquired the practices and took over the billing process experienced increased days in accounts receivable, terrible point-of-service collections, poor overall collection rates, and higher billing errors than those private practices had previously experienced.

The improved scale economies and the hospital billing expertise hospitals had hoped to leverage did not materialize. Even when the central billing function was controlled by a separate management services organization rather than the hospital central billing office (CBO), results were suboptimal when compared with effective private practice models. As the discussion at the retreat ensued, we documented a number of contributing factors that consistently surfaced:

1. Many of the errors dealt with by CBO personnel occurred at the reception desk in the medical practice network offices. Often, these errors where repeated, even after the receptionist was made aware of the issue.
2. Medical practice personnel were less likely to request co-payments and payment of other patient-due balances because money was now "their" (the CBO's) responsibility.
3. Because few electronic medical records were in use, the CBO staff did not have ready access to the information they needed to understand and correct a rejected claim. They were dependent on busy medical practice staff members who had access to the physician and the medical charts to research and forward information to the CBO.
4. Once the CBO took over billing, many medical practice staff members were delighted to divorce themselves from the billing and collections process and focus only on patient care and caring.

Much of this chapter was first published in B. Morton and M. Halley, "The Central Business/Processing Office," adapted, by permission, from *hfm* Magazine, March 2010, pages 36–40.

5. Constant finger pointing took place, with the CBO blaming the medical practices for errors and the practice staff insisting that the CBO team was not doing its job.

The Evolution of a Model

What came out of this afternoon exchange was the realization that structure had as much to do with the problem as the people involved. Structural questions included the following:

- What are the major causes of rejected claims, and where do those problems originate?
- Who possesses the information needed to yield a clean claim?
- Who should be responsible for each aspect of the revenue cycle process?
- Who can hold individuals accountable for each aspect of the revenue cycle process?
- Who has control over issuing credit to patients (e.g., those allowed to make payments over time)?
- Who has the best opportunity to collect cash from patients?
- What performance standard should be established for each step in the revenue cycle management process?

During our discussion it became clear that *access to patients and information* needed to be aligned with *accountability for performance measurement and reporting* at each step in the receivables management process. As subsequent experience has demonstrated, this alignment is even more important than the practice management software selected, the training provided, and other factors.

Our team started its search for a new approach to receivables management by listing each step in the revenue cycle process, as follows:

- Patient data gathering and verification (e.g., insurance and demographic data)
- Patient data entry
- Patient notice of co-payments
  —Point-of-service collection
  —Co-payments
- Balance due from the patient
- Fee ticket printing and attachment (paper systems)
- Coding of services (e.g., cognitive, procedural, ancillary)
- Documentation of services (e.g., physician, nurse, ancillary technician)
- Cashier station
  —Service data entry

  —Balance due from the patient
  —Credit extension/payment plans
- Claim audit
- Claim processing
  —Explanation-of-benefits data entry
  —Outstanding claims research
  —Rejected claims research
  —Contract management
- Patient statement processing
- Pre-collections notice processing
- Collections preview
- Pre-collections telephone contact
- Collections process
- Service termination

The team next asked "Who has the access to patients and their information necessary to complete the task most effectively and efficiently?" This exercise yielded the information shown in the first two columns of table 9-1.

As the information in this table materialized, it became clear why the concept of "central billing" did not work in a hospital-owned medical practice network setting. The central billing manager only had control of the information for *one-third* of the steps necessary to effectively manage the revenue cycle. In fact, the central billing manager only really controlled the processing function (e.g., claims and patient statements).

Since that day in Chicago, we have organized revenue cycle management according to our central processing office (CPO) model. The central processing approach places accountability for revenue cycle management with the practice manager in each practice setting. The CPO and the CPO manager provide processing support to help the practice manager accomplish his or her tasks. The practice manager is accountable to ensure compliance in steps 1–11 and 19–22 of the revenue cycle management process as enumerated in table 9-1.

The Central Processing Model in Practice

In practice, the benefits of the CPO model quickly become apparent. Front-office errors can be monitored and feedback sent to the practice manager, who can ensure that adequate training is provided, performance is measured, and those who consistently fail to perform their duties are replaced. The manager can also monitor how effectively (and with what frequency) the appointment clerk communicates co-payments and patient-due balances with those who call for appointments. Point-of-service collections can increase dramatically when receptionists and cashiers are held accountable daily to report their success at collecting over

Table 9-1. The Central Processing Office Model

Revenue Cycle Step	Access to Patients and Information	Performance Target
1. Patient data gathering and verification	Receptionist	98% clean claims (first run)
2. Patient data entry	Receptionist	98% clean claims (first run)
3. Patient notice of co-payments	Appointment desk	100% patients informed
4. Point-of-service collections—co-payments	Receptionist	95% of possible co-payments collected
5. Fee ticket printed and attached (paper systems)	Receptionist	100%
6. Coding for services	Physician or other provider	Ambulatory: 98% same day Surgery: 98% within 24 hours after operative report
7. Documentation of services	Physician or other provider	100% same day
8. Service data entry	Cashier	100% of charge tickets
9. Point-of-service collections---balance due	Cashier	Portion of balance due collected from 50% of patients presenting
10. Credit extension/payment plans	Cashier/office manager	100% of patient requests reviewed daily
11. Claims audit	Cashier	100% of charges pass system rules engine
12. Claims processing	Central processing	100% submission within 1 week of date of service
13. Explanation-of-benefits data entry	Central processing	95% of payments posted within 2 days of receipt
14. Outstanding claims research	Central processing	Claims worked within 5 business days on average by payer turnaround
15. Rejected claims research	Central processing	Claims worked within 2 business days of receipt
16. Payer contract review/ management	Central processing	Weekly reporting and follow-up within 10 business days
17. Patient statement processing	Central processing	100% of patients with balance receive statement monthly
18. Pre-collections notice processing	Central processing	100% qualifying patients receive each month
19. Collections pending list generation and review	Office manager or central processing	List reviewed by office within 5 business days of receipt from CPO
20. Pre-collections telephone contact	Office manager and physician	100% of patients contacted by office prior to submission to collection agency (5 business days to connect)
21. Collections process	Outside vendor	Monthly submission of 98% of qualifying patients
22. Service termination	Office manager and physician	Case-by-case review with office manager and physician within 5 business days of receipt from CPO

the counter, which is the most efficient (least costly) and most effective way to collect payments. The CPO supports the practice manager in all these activities by providing training in the use of the practice management software and providing feedback on rejected or denied claims by reason.

Coding experts have long recommended that physicians and others providing the services are in the best position to identify the procedure and diagnosis codes and to document the services performed. Ideally, the cashier is a second set of experienced eyes working with the practice management software and electronic medical record to ensure a clean claim. If questions arise, the cashier is often able to preempt problems by communicating with the physician. The practice manager works with the physicians to monitor the coding index (the number of work relative value units divided by the number of patient visits) by provider each month.

The CPO model supports effective coding and documentation by employing one or more coding experts who provide at least annual training updates, a coding help desk (used most often by the cashier), and quarterly audits of charts for each physician, with follow-up training provided individually. Importantly, the CPO also documents coding- and documentation-related reasons for denied claims; it feeds that information back to the practice manager and the physicians through the coding expert.

In addition to having expertise in coding and documentation and providing training for and maintenance of the practice management system, the CPO is the expert insurance claims processor. The CPO team members develop expertise in managing claims according to payer contract. They deal with claims that are outstanding to speed up processing and quickly resolve denials. The CPO produces patient statements monthly or more frequently based on date of last activity. It usually supports the pre-collections process by sending to patients approved dunning notices and to each POC a recommended list of patients whose delinquency merits a more formal collections process and service termination. The practice manager and physicians should review and approve all such hard collections/terminations.

In addition, as part of the pre-collections process we recommend that the practice manager make telephone contact with all patients/guarantors prior to formal collections and service termination procedures. Obviously, if errors (which usually occur on the front end of the revenue cycle management process) can be solved at their source through training, measurement, and proper accountability, CPO team members will have more time to devote to managing claims and payers.

Performance Measures

Wise managers know that anything they measure improves. Changing the structure of the revenue cycle management process to better align access to patients and information with accountability for results can dramatically improve those results. But structural change alone is not enough to guarantee optimum performance. If the organization fails to measure performance at *every step* of the revenue cycle management process, its outcomes will be suboptimal because failure at any step can derail or delay the entire process.

Experience has shown that the party responsible for each step is the best one to measure and personally report those results, even if the practice management system allows the practice manager and the CPO manager to gather performance data themselves. That daily or weekly "return and report" by each incumbent gives the manager an opportunity to motivate improved performance, understand the barriers to performance, identify training opportunities, and improve processes or support systems.

Some suggested measures for each step in the revenue cycle management process are included in the third column of table 9-1.

Managing Payments

As indicated earlier, the least expensive way to collect medical practice fees for services rendered is at the point of service. An effective point-of-service (POS) collections process starts with setting this expectation in the minds of new and established patients. A well-written letter of explanation inviting patients to "help us keep our costs down" and a blurb in the patient brochure are great ways to begin setting that expectation.

The appointment clerk politely reminding patients about their co-payment and balance due is another huge help in promoting POS collections. Patients arrive at the practice expecting to make a payment or co-payment, reducing the chance for any embarrassment. The collection of co-payments before the day's visit by an effective receptionist and collection of patient-due balances after the patient encounter by a skilled cashier will have a tremendous influence on reducing the costs of collecting fees and reducing bad debt write-offs.

The most effective cashiers we know consider it their mission to "help you get us paid." They view themselves as patient advocates, helping patients/customers sort out and understand insurance and private balances. They are comfortable asking for payment of all or a portion of the current or previously outstanding amounts. Some use a carefully crafted script in their discussions; others just seem to have a knack for encouraging patients to turn over money and feel good about it.

Despite a sound process and the best efforts of the POS team, most medical practices usually end up with active patients who have outstanding balances after insurance companies have paid their share of the bill. Most do not charge interest on those outstanding balances but are, by default, still offering credit. In fact, while most surgery practices ultimately achieve a zero balance, many primary care practices and those that treat chronic disease have active patients whose long-standing balances look a lot like revolving credit, moving up and down over time.

By definition, allowing patients to pay over time, with or without charging interest on the outstanding balance, constitutes an extension of credit. As a result, even small medical practices become subject to regulations governing credit extension. Compliance with these regulations is often ignored by private practices simply because they are unaware of their obligations. Such ignorance, however, is increasingly risky and could be costly in terms of stiff fines for each violation.

Hospital-owned network executives should be conscious of the regulations governing covered patient accounts, including required patient notifications, identity theft protections, truth-in-lending requirements (for practices that charge interest on unpaid balances), billing cycle rules, and telephone collections rules. Both federal regulations and state laws apply to credit extension. Readers are encouraged to consult with local legal counsel to ensure that their revenue cycle management process is compliant. The rules identified should become part of the medical practice network compliance manual.

Collections methods employed by hospitals have received some negative press in the past few years. A few hospitals and health systems have been accused of heartless attitudes and ruthless methods in pursuing collections efforts. The accusers are always quick to point out the fact that such facilities are "not-for-profit" and therefore have an obligation to see all those who present for services regardless of their ability (or even willingness) to pay.

Leaving the ethical debate to experts in that arena, the business fact remains that some patients served in hospitals and hospital-owned practices find themselves in challenging financial straits. Several of our clients have established charity care policies that provide graduated payment scales or even free care to those who are truly needy, as determined by household income levels. Establishing such a policy is a great help to cashiers and office managers when they encounter someone who is truly needy, and they can offer assistance accordingly to those who qualify.

Training—It's Mission Critical

Combine the complexity of medical practice insurance and billing, the challenges of learning a practice management system, employee turnover, and no accountability at the front desk, and the importance of training becomes clear. Failure to measure—or worse, ignore—the financial results over several months because the amounts are small when compared with hospital receivables will result in an accounts receivable nightmare. Once structural problems have been corrected and performance measures are put in place, ongoing employee training becomes mission critical. In fact, the more practice employees know about insurance plans, procedure and diagnosis coding, and the practice management system, the more effective and efficient will be the revenue cycle management process.

In our experience, the CPO should be the source of training and support for the entire revenue cycle management process. Depending on the size of the physician network, the CPO manager should hire one or more skilled trainers for the revenue cycle management process, insurance billing requirements, the practice management system, and procedure coding and documentation. Formal training classes should be available on a continual basis for new hires, and annual updates should be required for established employees.

Even those who think they know the process and systems should be required to attend annual updates. Those established employees who have demonstrated their capabilities on the job may even be asked to teach, under the guidance of the training manager. Such assignments are often highly motivational for the instructors and most helpful for the attendees, who benefit from those with real-world, real-time experience. The better the training, the better will be compliance with correct operating principles and the more effective will be the entire revenue cycle management process.

The Practice Management System

Chapter 10 focuses on information technology and the planning, selection, and installation of practice management (PM) and electronic medical records systems. For our discussion here, the PM system must support the revenue cycle management process in two ways. First, it must have the software capabilities and modules necessary to support the CPO process at every step, from POS collections to claims scrubbers, from claims processing to payer contract management. Second, the PM system must be installed with the CPO process in mind so that definitions, permissions, input screens, information inquiry, and training are aligned with the distributed approach.

Obviously, physician networks should select one and only one practice management system to support their revenue cycle management process. Allowing individual practices to maintain their software as a term of practice acquisition or in order to avoid additional capital investment can be the death knell for effective and efficient receivables management. The right software package supports not only the revenue cycle process itself but also individual accountability for effective management of the process.

Results from the Central Processing Model

The results of the transition from a traditional central billing to a central processing revenue cycle management model can be significant. We have seen multiple clients with more than 100 days in accounts receivable experience a decrease to forty days or less, accompanied by increased collections as a percentage of charges. Our CPO clients have seen practice managers take the reins and dramatically reduce errors on the front end of the process. CPO managers are delighted to be accountable and focus only on those portions of the revenue cycle management process within their control. The finger pointing is a distant memory, and the bottom line results are obvious.

A CPO approach usually requires fewer staff than a traditional CBO model. Consequently, the cost of the CPO approach is lower. This phenomenon occurs for two reasons. First, POS collections increase in the practices, requiring less statement processing and private pay management on the back end. Second, far less rework occurs throughout the process because roles/functions and accountability for results are aligned; hence the work is correct the first time.

Summary

While practice management systems do have a great influence on the success of the revenue cycle management processes, developing a proper structure that aligns *access to information and patients* with *accountability for performance measurement and reporting* has an even more dramatic effect on overall performance. The transition process includes additional training and accountability for medical practice managers and staff, but their work load remains essentially the same with improved accuracy and less rework for the entire process.

This chapter highlights the critical need for continuous training, even once the CPO model is well ingrained. The central processing model helps ensure the continued success of the medical practices served by maximizing the dollars collected and minimizing the costs of doing so.

CHAPTER 10

Information Technology

Chapter 7 discusses the concept that people are an organization's most valuable asset. It is through people that we provide our high-quality care in a caring manner. Chapter 8 presents ways to maximize the productivity of people: We discussed the concept of highest and best-use staffing, whereby people in primary roles do what they are best trained and qualified to do and delegate the balance of their work to people in secondary roles. This chapter focuses on information as the great enabler of quality and productivity leading to operational and financial viability.

Physicians, other providers, management, and support staff—people—represent 70 to 80 percent of the cost structure of most medical practices. Information about patients, guarantors, payer plans, eligibility, clinical services, insurance claims, patient-due balances, referrals, cash collections, payroll costs, and much, much more facilitates and is evidence of their work. Technology has provided us with the ability to gather, store, manipulate, use, and communicate information more effectively and efficiently than ever before. However, the use of technology is no guarantee that information will flow effectively or efficiently. In fact, poorly designed software, inadequately configured and improperly applied to broken processes, produces a bigger mess quicker than no technology at all, reducing both the efficiency and the effectiveness of our most costly human resources and potentially reducing clinical and service outcomes.

New technology can enhance our ability to treat disease, automate processes to eliminate variability, reduce cost, dramatically improve productivity, identify trends and potential problems, and otherwise benefit humankind. In each of these situations, technology is the tool, not the master. The same principle applies to information technology (IT). Information technology is that set of tools that facilitates the flow of information so that individuals and organizations can achieve their potential. In order to be effective, technology must facilitate the flow of information in support of operational processes that allow people to perform their work.

Physicians and support staff need to drive the selection and use of technology tools in medical practice networks. These decisions are operational in nature, to be made by those providing the medical services rather than be driven by a hospital IT department agenda. While an IT department must be involved in technology decisions, its members should serve as technology experts and facilitators, not as the operational decision makers.

Applied Information Technology

Like any new technology, information technology should be acquired and implemented to achieve specific objectives. Ideally, objectives related to needs and requirements are understood and documented before the search for technology solutions commences. As with all key decisions made in a medical practice network, the application of technology should be measured against all four critical success filters. That is, does the proposed information technology solution:

1. Maintain or enhance clinical quality as defined by the practice physicians?
2. Maintain or enhance service quality as defined by the patients and their referring physicians?
3. Maintain or enhance physician (and staff) productivity?
4. Maintain or enhance operational or financial viability?

The application of information technology presents an opportunity to review operational objectives, performance expectations, existing systems, and current processes with an eye toward targeted performance improvement. Properly designed IT applications facilitate best practices found in similar settings rather than simply automating existing processes. Proper selection of IT application software is based on the needs and objectives of the particular medical practice network. Software selection should not be based on the hospital platform just because the current hospital vendor has a medical practice application as a sideline. Any application software decision should be based on an independent evaluation that includes functional requirements and needs, that considers multiple vendors (with no pre-selection determined by hospital incumbent software), and that is based on a vendor's/solution's respective abilities to meet the physician network's objectives.

Within regulatory constraints, it is usually a business imperative that data captured in one system can be passed to, and used by, other software systems without manual intervention. In the past, many software decisions were based on the assumption that using two software packages offered by the same vendor would ensure a flawless data flow. In fact, however, some purchasers have been sorely disappointed when data flow was far from perfect. Because many software vendors purchase applications from other companies, one cannot assume that two products from the same vendor will use data in a seamless fashion. On the other hand, in today's world of sophisticated interfaces, the ability of one application to "talk to" another virtually eliminates the incompatibility argument. With proper attention to mapping data and applying data validation/edit rules, interoperability can usually be achieved and is no longer a limiting factor in software decisions.

Making the best decision for each business unit (e.g., hospital, medical practices) based on the rules for success in that unit is an increasingly compelling objective. Rather than selecting a single solution from a single vendor that may have a great practice management system and a fair electronic medical record (EMR) (or vice versa), a physician network may be better served by selecting the best of breed for each application and dealing with the interfacing issues.

Mission-Critical Applications

Two applications are mission critical for a medical practice network. The first is the practice management (PM) system that supports practice operations from the appointment schedule and patient registration to coding and billing for services. Virtually every medical practice has automated its practice management system during the past thirty years. The second critical application is the EMR, sometimes called the electronic health record. The automation of these clinical records has been and still is a key political agenda, the argument of which is that digitizing records will reduce costs, eliminate medical errors, and improve clinical outcomes. Although many health systems, hospitals, and larger practices have installed a partial or full EMR, most small, independent practices have not implemented any form of electronic record technology. Many top hospital-based EMRs are fully integrated with their own practice management system, which, again, may or may not meet the needs of a particular physician network organization.

As a best practice, both of these mission-critical applications should be standardized across a hospital-owned medical practice network. The decision making around both critical software systems needs to engage clinicians, practice operations management, and support staff users, who become the *primary drivers* of the ultimate solution. Information technology department experts should provide support and counsel in documenting infrastructure criteria (hardware, bandwidth, security, capacity, volumes, backup, redundancy, and so forth) and should participate as part of a team in the evaluation of multiple software candidates; the selection and contracting process; the configuration, data conversion, and installation process; and, very importantly, the assurance that adequate ongoing training will be offered and application and hardware support will be provided.

The selection and implementation of these critical applications is not the place to skimp on investment. There are no shortcuts, and "cheaper" is not necessarily better. Failure to select, configure, and properly implement IT turns this enabler into a huge disabler, damaging clinical quality, service quality, productivity, and operational and financial viability (not to mention creating tremendous frustration for the people involved, including the customer). The costs of these consequences are difficult to quantify, but a few moments spent in a practice that made the wrong choice will convince any skeptic that those consequent costs easily eclipse the additional dollars necessary to make the right decision in the first place, pay for the extra interface, contract for the extra training, and sponsor additional IT staff or the vendor contract to properly support the application(s).

Selecting Mission-Critical Applications

The selection process for mission-critical applications includes the following steps:

- Engaging the project team
- Determining system requirements
- Soliciting proposals from potential vendors
- Evaluating request for proposal (RFP) responses to choose the more viable contenders
- Viewing and scoring vendor demonstrations to make a first cut
- Inviting the better vendors to a call-back round of demonstrations
- Developing a final list of the best vendors
- Negotiating a contract with the finalists
- Assembling an implementation team

The Project Team

It has been said that people do not buy in to a decision because they are involved; they buy in because they understand.[1] I cannot think of a more significant success factor in organizational decision making. Engaging a cross-functional team from different practices in a network is essential to identify needs, review options, select software, and plan implementation. Because few software decisions (or any decisions, for that matter) are perfect, engaging credible participants in the selection process is critical to making the best decision and to acceptance of that decision by the organization.

Project team members will likely include a cross-section of job functions affecting or affected by the software decision, a cross-section of practices and specialties, hospital support departments/experts, and management. Ideally, the project team includes a credible clinical champion whose influence and encouragement will be felt by others during the education and implementation process. For example, a strong and credible physician champion can go a long way toward ameliorating the fears of fellow physicians facing the implementation of an EMR.

Determining System Requirements

Experts agree that the more time spent understanding and thoroughly defining the needs, wants, and priorities of those most affected by the software, the more successful will be the process of selection and conversion. A properly designed project team will help identify those needs, wants, and priorities. Even this select group, however, should not operate in a vacuum. Because most networks include multiple locations, each facing varying challenges, keeping the entire organization apprised of the developing functional requirements list will pay huge dividends during the implementation process.

The list of functional requirements usually includes certain *non-negotiable* capabilities, which should clearly be identified for review within the organization and for potential vendors. Those critical elements become the minimum standards that vendors must address to even be considered by the project team. These elements will form the basis of the RFP, discussed later in this chapter.

The next tier of requirements will include those *desired* capabilities that would be nice to have but are not considered essential to functionality in the setting. We encourage our clients to prioritize and weight this list of options from most useful to least significant. Because options sometimes complicate matters or increase costs, they should be weighed against their potential value in the network setting. For example, requirements might be categorized as:

A Non-negotiable/required
B Strongly desired (may be improvements from the status quo)
C Nice to have/optional

Appendix I presents a list of potential requirement considerations for mission-critical application selection. This list is not exhaustive but is provided to elicit ideas from project team members. Whether the organization is replacing either or both mission-critical systems, adding an EMR for the first time, or considering an integrated package or separate systems, many of these components apply to the decision making.

The Request for Proposal

If you take your RFP seriously, your serious vendors will do the same. As one who has developed and responded to RFPs, I can witness that the more time you take to clearly define your requirements and organize them effectively, the more useful will be the vendor responses—at least those you should spend time evaluating.

The RFP should include your critical functional elements, those non-negotiable capabilities that will separate out viable contenders from those pursuing a long shot. These minimal capabilities should be front and center in the RFP responses so you can quickly eliminate those who do not qualify. The RFP should also include those additional options you would like to consider. We recommended sharing this option list, priorities, and weighting with the vendors so they know how to respond and price their proposals. Importantly, we recommend that you provide adequate time for your vendors to offer a thoughtful response to your RFP. You should offer the vendor at least as much time to respond as it took your project team to create and approve the RFP (assuming your team is reasonably efficient).

We recommend that, while the RFP is being written, members of the project team pre-screen potential vendors to develop a qualified list of those to whom you will send your completed request. We suggest that they interview several professional colleagues to assess their experience with the PM and EMR solutions and vendors they have selected or even rejected. In our experience, the satisfactory vendors will quickly rise to the top in multiple settings. More importantly, colleagues will usually share any train wrecks they have experienced (although some executives may be contractually bound not to share their experience, which should, of course, be a red flag in itself). We recommend that, as qualified vendors surface, project team members attend available conferences, exhibits, and demonstrations to get a feel for the systems and people representing the vendors. Once a pre-screened vendor list has been developed, the completed RFP can be distributed to each listed vendor.

RFP Evaluation

We recommend that, based on the criteria identified in the RFP, the project team develop, in advance, an objective RFP score sheet for assessing the responses that includes a section for subjective comments. Several types of score sheets should be used during the evaluation process. They provide a quantifiable method to evaluate vendors. The scores resulting from the RFP review will determine which vendors are invited to demonstrate their software to the project team. We often see between four and ten vendors invited to this initial screening, who visit at their own expense. We are also comfortable letting the vendors know who else will be sharing the demonstration stage.

First-Cut Demonstrations

The initial screening, or first-cut demonstrations (demos), will likely be canned presentations highlighting the features of the respective packages. As with the RFP evaluation process, we recommend the development of a first-cut demo score sheet for each project team member to complete after each vendor's demonstration. Team member impressions of the strengths and weaknesses of each vendor will be most useful when compared with one another. After these initial demonstrations are complete, we engage project team members in explaining why they scored each vendor as they did, which often yields new insights that can be applied to subsequent evaluation. The scores and discussion will usually weed out all but the few vendors that come closest to addressing all of the required criteria and many desired options.

Call-Back Demonstrations

After the first-cut demonstrations, those two to four vendors with the best scores should be invited to participate in call-back demonstrations. The call-back invitation will include the network's request for a more detailed supplemental response, to be returned prior to the vendors' final presentation, as well as the work flow script (described later in this section), which vendors must use during their call-back demonstrations. If you included all of the following components in your RFP, there may be no need for a supplemental response. However, we usually recommend that you require these components only of those vendors that make the initial cut.

THE SUPPLEMENTAL RESPONSE

The supplemental response should include topics such as the following:

- *Standards.* How does the software currently meet regulatory requirements such as the Health Insurance Portability and Accountability Act and accreditation standards such as the Certification Commission for Healthcare Information Technology? What is the vendor's track record and commitment to meeting these changing requirements?
- *Meaningful use.* How does the software meet the definition of meaningful use as currently promulgated?
- *Data conversion.* What is the vendor's process, and what have been the outcomes of previous data conversions? What is its experience converting data from our current systems (PM and/or EMR)?
- *Data interface.* What is the vendor's experience with moving data among the (1) PM application, (2) EMR application, and (3) hospital EMR, as appropriate?
- *Data configuration.* What is the vendor's process for leading an organization through the many edits, rules, roles, and work flow processes that must be determined in order to promote a successful implementation?
- *Installation process.* What is the vendor's process for software installation, and what have been the outcomes of previous installations?
- *Training and documentation.* What is the vendor's initial training process? What are the measures and minimum competencies for users, and how successful have its training processes been in achieving those competencies? What documentation is available to users, "super users," and local IT support staff? What supplemental training is available?
- *Maintenance and support.* What ongoing maintenance, training, and support are available directly from the vendor for users, and what support would be available to the internal IT experts?
- *Platform.* Is the system centralized on hardware at the organization's location, or is it hosted at the vendor's data center and accessed via the

Internet? Why has the vendor chosen this platform? Why is this platform appropriate for your network?

- *Company information.* Company information should include such factors as time in the business, fiscal strength, management capabilities, the age of the product, the number of dedicated developers and annual turnover, the number of dedicated support staff members and annual turnover, help desk staffing and support hours, choices in support level, and the profile of its installed customer base.
- *References.* Provide references for similar system/network/medical specialty installations, as well as those that have similar data interfaces.
- *Development process.* What is the vendor's product development timetable? (For example, what is the schedule for new releases, and how does the vendor handle unscheduled updates?) How do new releases accommodate any customized components? How mature is the current product? What version? Is the vendor the original developer? If not, from whom did it buy the product? What is the plan for future product evolution and the schedule for implementing enhancements?
- *Development platform.* What is the database engine and the programming language? Is it open or proprietary? What peripherals and clinical devices are supported by the software to improve clinical and business productivity? What is the vendor's connection with user groups to identify best practices?
- *Costs.* How will the initial costs be determined for the items listed below?
  —Software (licensure)
  —Data conversion
  —Data interface
  —Customizations
  —Installation
  —Initial training
  —Maintenance and upgrades
  —Technical support
  How will those costs be determined after year 1? What impact will additional users have on those costs, and at what thresholds?
- *Strengths and weaknesses.* Each vendor should be asked to assess the strengths and weaknesses of its product against those of the other call-back vendors in terms of capabilities.

A supplemental response score sheet should be developed to evaluate each vendor's responses. Any item requiring clarification can be pursued at the end of the vendor's call-back demonstration. The supplemental response is used to delve "behind the scenes" to components that are not obvious to the typical user. It facilitates assessment of the functionality and stability of the software. "Pretty screens" are of little use if database management, maintenance, security, and so forth are overly complex or inadequate.

Call-back demonstrations should be driven by the project team and should be specific to your network and situation. These final demonstrations are intended to broaden the evaluation process to users beyond the project team. These call-back demos (usually multiple sessions for each vendor/application) should be scheduled at times that do not conflict with physicians seeing patients. Nursing staff, receptionists, appointment clerks, billing staff, management, and others should be well represented in this final evaluation. Again, involvement in the decision-making process is not enough. Broad understanding of the decision will facilitate its acceptance and subsequent implementation.

THE WORK FLOW SCRIPT

Call-back demonstrations should be based on a work flow script that the project team develops. The work flow script should detail the work flow the team would like to see demonstrated, based on your specific operational requirements.

Be sure to incorporate into the script typical scenarios encountered in your practices, as well as those that are currently a challenge. For example, the practice management software and installation should be able to support the central processing office approach to revenue cycle management. The EMR software should be able to support not only high-quality clinical requirements but also quality service, physician productivity, and financial and operational viability.

The script should include time for the vendor to create a report "real time" during the demonstration. For example, the team will pose a functional question and have the vendor demonstrate how quickly/easily it can produce a view/report to answer the question. The vendor should *not* be given this question in advance.

THE CALL-BACK DEMO SCORE SHEET

The call-back demo score sheet should include all components identified in the work flow script. Great care should be taken to work with users in designing the scoring tool for physicians and staff. That tool will likely include issues affecting their work lives, such as ease and efficiency of software use, friendliness of screens, ease of data entry, usefulness of prompts, access to information, "speed sets" to facilitate documentation, the presence and usefulness of a report writer (having the vendor create a report on-site), the availability of training materials, and other operational factors. Users will naturally be concerned about how intuitive each system might be. As with all decisions, maintaining or enhancing clinical quality, service quality, productivity, and operational and financial viability should be key evaluative filters included in the score sheet.

The call-back demo score sheet must be completed by every participant at the end of each vendor's call-back demo (before they leave the demo). "Every participant" includes all physicians, clinical staff, administrative staff, project team, managers, the hospital IT department, and others involved with the system. If these evaluation sheets are not turned in before participants leave the demo, not only will your return rate greatly diminish but participants will have difficulty remembering who did what in which demo; as a result, findings will become blurred and inaccurate.

Final List of Vendors

Once the call-back demonstrations are complete and the call-back demo score sheets evaluated, the project team should develop the final list of vendors that appear to meet all of the organization's requirements. On occasion, a single vendor will rise head and shoulders above the rest, making the decision easy. More often, however, two or three vendors will come close to meeting your needs, wants, and priorities, but none will fit your organization perfectly. It is desirable to have at least two vendors in this category, which will improve your negotiating position.

The project team needs to evaluate these finalists side by side, comparing the pros and cons in ways that will be understood by the various internal stakeholders who will be affected by the team's final software recommendation. This comparison will include detailed reference checks covering many of the topics previously discussed. The project team and others should definitely conduct site visits to organizations that have been using the candidate application for at least six months (a year or more is preferable) to observe how the system functions in daily operations. Each site visit should include interviews with site managers, physicians, support staff, and IT staff to discuss their experience with the implementation process, functionality, training, maintenance, and so forth. It must be stressed that *no application should be selected* without seeing it in use at another organization. Group members should debrief and document their experience at each site.

Contract Negotiations

The vendor finalists should each have the opportunity to submit their best price and terms the first time. Again, this pricing should include not only the purchase/installation costs but also the costs during out years (years 2 through 5). Ongoing maintenance, support, upgrade, and customization costs can often be as great as or greater than the initial purchase cost. The project team should then evaluate the pricing and terms against the value they perceive. A software purchase is a long-term partnership with the selected vendor, and it is in your best interest to be a good customer. We recommend that our clients avoid the "nickel and dime" game—squeezing the last $1,000 out of the deal. Make sure that the vendor makes a reasonable profit so your installation will continue to be of interest as a client. Certainly, we recommend questioning terms or pricing that appear to be outliers—most vendors appreciate the opportunity to know where they can look to sharpen their proposal, but encourage them to offer their best deal the first time and then honor that response. In addition, be sure to review a vendor's contract for performance standards and service-level commitments, as well as a defined process for retaining and accessing your organization's data in the event of contract termination.

Once the final proposals, pricing, and terms have been received, the project team evaluates the options and selects a recommended system and vendor for consideration by the decision maker. Again, we recommend that the project team document the key factors driving the ultimate selection. This documentation will be a key part of the communication process as the new system is announced and installed.

The Implementation Team

Selecting the application is only the beginning of an intensive process. Once the selection has been made, an implementation team must be assembled to develop an implementation plan and drive it to completion. The implementation team must include a cross-section of clinical, administrative, and technical personnel.

This step provides a golden opportunity to improve work flow processes in the practices, as opposed to "automating broken processes." The time and attention given to incorporating best practices and improved processes will be exponentially rewarded. While the following list is not inclusive, it is representative of the variety and types of issues the implementation team will need to address:

- *Roles.* Determine which roles or jobs need access to which software modules or menu items, as well as the extent of that access. Develop a matrix of security clearance, access, and constraints (e.g., read-only access versus editing rights).
- *Rules.* Document appropriate work flow, processes, and procedures that must be supported by the software.
- *Data conversion and mapping.* Understand which data from the current system will be transferred to the new system and how it will be mapped to appropriate fields or files in the new application (applies only if there is an existing system).
- *Data edits.* Document the required fields, acceptable values, and drop-down lists to support/edit data entry by users.
- *Configuration.* Develop supportive menus and selection lists for ease of access by users.
- *Users.* Identify specific users according to their roles to determine their permissions, required training, and minimum competencies before the system goes live.

- *Paper records.* Identify paper records from external sources and how they will be accommodated in the new system.
- *Charting.* Identify charting options and requirements based on each physician's and mid-level provider's preference (e.g., voice, keyboard, speed sets).
- *Training.* Identify training requirements by role/job. Define the initial and ongoing training process, including local trainers, help desk support, and super users. Define training locations (e.g., practice site or centralized training room).
- *Testing.* Identify the process for testing data integrity, appropriate work flow, software interfaces, supporting modules, and the system as a whole.
- *Benchmark.* Document and compare anticipated and actual system performance and capacity, with particular emphasis on network throughput (whether on a local central processor or by using the Internet to access an off-site hosted system).
- *Redundancy.* Determine the required bandwidth as well as redundant servers and computers to ensure the organization's ability to survive short-term interruptions in power, Internet access, and so forth.
- *Disaster recovery.* Identify the process for minimum functionality in case of PM or EMR unavailability or failure due to a major disaster.

Summary

The right information technology solution is the great enabler of high-quality care and caring. It also supports provider productivity and operational and financial viability. The wrong IT solution or a poorly implemented solution can damage quality and productivity beyond repair in terms of service disruption and costs. Consequently, great care must be taken in the selection and implementation of practice management and electronic medical record software across a medical practice network. Information technology solutions are operations decisions rather than IT decisions and require the involvement of end users to ensure the right choice is made. Effective installation/implementation supports high clinical quality, service quality, physician productivity, operational viability, and financial performance.

Reference

1. Kerry Patterson, Joseph Grenny, Ron McMillan, and Al Switzler, *Crucial Conversations: Tools for Talking When the Stakes Are High,* 23 (New York: McGraw-Hill, 2002).

CHAPTER 11

Facilities and Equipment

Many hospital executives have applied the same "build it and they will come" model used over the years in hospital settings to their hospital-owned medical practices. Some have invested millions in new campus-based and off-campus medical office buildings or collaborated with developers and signed long-term leases. The new facilities are usually beautifully designed and often have centralized laboratory and imaging services staffed by the hospital.

Thinking strategically, hospital strategists develop facilities that will accommodate potential growth, perhaps housing several practices. The buildings frequently include 10,000 to 50,000 square feet or more of usable space. The lease costs range from $20 to $30 per square foot, sometimes double what private practices pay for office space in the same markets.

Market Share and Other Considerations

Perhaps nothing at all is wrong with the additional medical office space. However, too often, facility sponsors fail to consider the following:

- Market share
- Market saturation
- Lease cost
- Ancillary services
- Specialty mix
- The shower stall
- Empty space

Market Share

The primary focus of capital expenditures should be capturing market share rather than adding bricks and mortar. Placing the organization's logo on multiple buildings does little to attract patients to primary care physicians or to promote referrals to specialists. Investing in properly located primary care practices and attracting the resulting market share to the capital-generating engine ensures adequate capital to continue growing the business.

On one occasion, for example, we assisted a large, multi-location, multispecialty group that was being courted by two competing local health systems, each of which wanted to pursue a stronger affiliation. Both local systems employed primary care physicians who provided referrals to our specialty-dominated medical practice client. The risk inherent in such a decision was significant for the medical group, and its decision would have potentially significant implications for each health system.

After much debate and discussion, we presented slides documenting the locations of the two competing hospital-owned primary care networks. One of the competing systems had located its employed primary care physicians on or near its hospital campuses. The other system had distributed its primary care network throughout the region. Understanding how our Mrs. Smith, introduced in chapter 5, makes her primary care physician decisions, the second, neighborhood approach was much more appealing to the multispecialty group as it considered which local health system had the sustainable strategic advantage.

Market Saturation

Developers focus on filling medical office space and often fail to consider the neighborhood's saturation point—particularly for primary care practices. Moving established primary care practices located within a ten-minute drive into the new space may make sense if the physicians support the consolidation effort as a platform for creating a group practice. However, locating physicians within the same space in a building does not necessarily yield an integrated group. It is highly unlikely that consolidation will yield any net cost savings even if the new group is able to take advantage of some limited economies of scale. Worse, if the consolidated group loses a multi-neighborhood location advantage to competitors, the new group practice may struggle to remain viable in the future.

Similarly, co-locating specialty practices in close physical proximity to primary care practices does not necessarily yield more referrals to those specialists. Issues of appointment access, relationship and communication with the primary care physician (PCP), and previous patient experience have much more to do with patient referrals than whether or not the specialist is located down the hall or on a different floor in the medical office building (MOB) or ambulatory care center.

Lease Cost

The cost of newly built space is often double that which private practicing physicians pay for existing space in the same market. Such costs are hard to justify. The new space is unquestionably beautiful and comfortable, but beauty and comfort are not significant factors in attracting or retaining market share in the form of patient or primary care referrals. Patients and physicians are just as happy with their service provided in properly located, well-equipped, pleasantly appointed space at half the price per square foot. We encourage our hospital clients to clean up existing space. Elbow grease, a can of paint, new carpet, new furnishings, new plants, and artwork can revitalize an older facility in the right neighborhood. If either the space or location is inadequate, we encourage our clients to use less expensive storefront space in strip malls where successful retailers are located.

Clearly, having certain invasive specialties located in an attached medical office building with easy access to hospital operating suites and procedure rooms does provide value. These specialists and their patients actually use the hospital and its facilities. Specialists may also be in a better financial position to justify the premium cost per square foot.

Ancillary Services

As indicated earlier, particularly in ambulatory settings away from the hospital campus, customers prefer to receive common ancillary services—laboratory, imaging, screening, and so forth—right in their doctor's office.

Certainly, the opportunity to access more advanced imaging services without having to go to the hospital campus would be appreciated by those few patients who need an MRI (magnetic resonance imaging) or a CT (computed tomography) scan, but these represent a relatively small percentage of referrals for most primary care and for many specialty practices.

As with the specialty physician mix, discussed below, we recommend that our clients first capture and then carefully assess the market share in primary care practices. Based on the needs of the PCPs and their patients, facilities and equipment to serve those needs can then be developed to enhance physician and patient satisfaction and convenience.

Specialty Mix

Specialty physicians have two critical customers. The most important is the referring physician, who will be responsible for future referrals. The second most important customer is Mrs. Smith, whose experience with the specialist and his or her support staff will certainly be communicated to the referring physician and will affect future referrals. Facility location and design decisions for a specialty practice should take into account the four critical success filters discussed throughout the book: clinical quality, service quality, physician productivity, and operational and financial viability. From the hospital's perspective, specialty recruitment and location decisions are a function of service line strategies, including attracting market share to those service lines through its affiliated physician specialists.

Positioning the right specialist in a rural community to improve access and communication with local referring physicians and to support the local community hospital is a proven method for attracting tertiary business. Those decisions are frequently based on business already flowing from the outlying community. Similar positioning strategies can be implemented in a hospital's primary service area. For example, tracking referrals from primary care providers in one quadrant of the community may indicate the need for a cardiology practice; an ear, nose, and throat practice; an orthopedic practice; or others in that area to improve access for patients and communication with referring physicians.

If the specialist will be serving a larger primary care practice, he or she should consider rotating through the PCP practice and contributing to overhead expenses at fair market value. If the specialty practice will serve several primary care practices (owned or independent practices), planners should select a central location for the specialty practice so that referring physicians do not perceive they will lose any patients they refer to the specialist. Laboratory, imaging, and procedural services can be made available to those specialty physicians and their patients, as discussed above.

Some of our clients have used the traditional "hot suite" with tremendous success. In local or regional markets where patient referrals are not adequate to support one or more full-time specialty physicians, developers can establish a shared suite with a receptionist and telephone line(s) to support appointment scheduling for one or more rotating specialists. Some hot suites provide clinical support staff, ancillary services, and even billing and collections services for specialists who participate.

The Shower Stall

Over the years, we have found many constructed—but never used—shower stalls in new facilities. In almost every case, their tiled surfaces have become very expensive storage closets and monuments to a physician's grand design or New Year's resolution that had little to do with the business at hand. "Buy 'em a gym pass" is our mantra in addressing the argument.

Facility design should focus on the four critical success filters reiterated above. Special care should be taken to ensure that the productivity zone, as described in chapter 8, is designed to facilitate high productivity and accommodate high volume. Ancillary services should be conveniently located to ensure that they support productivity rather than becoming a bottleneck, on even the busy days. The design of the reception area should include comfortable furnishings and should facilitate the receptionist's role in monitoring the reception room like a lifeguard watching those bobbing heads in the pool.

Empty Space

We understand the wisdom of developing space for future expansion. We also see how frustrating it is for two new physicians to "rattle around" in 15,000 square feet as they try to build new practices. The impact of that extra space on the income statement can be disheartening for physicians and staff concerned with achieving practice viability—and they all should be concerned about meeting that critical target over time.

We recommend using two net income lines on the hospital-owned medical practice income statements, regardless of specialty.[1] Net income line one (net one) reflects all the revenues and only those expenses that would be found in a small group private practice (e.g., office manager, billing costs). Net income line two (net two) reflects the additional expenses found in a large hospital-owned network (e.g., a network executive, region managers). Using this method, empty office space is placed in the net two category as a strategic expense not associated with current practice operations. (The principles of net one and net two income lines are discussed further in chapter 12.)

Big Box or Small Box?

In a number of markets around the United States, hospital executives are developing large ambulatory care centers around their primary service areas. Square footage, services available, and strategic purposes for these facilities vary. Some are built on several acres as the foundation for a campus model that may ultimately include additional or replacement beds. Others include an outpatient surgery center to relieve an overcrowded hospital campus and operating rooms. Some are strictly focused on ambulatory services and on providing convenient primary care, specialty care, and ancillary services to growing/evolving communities. Some are built with the intent to achieve certain economies of scale. Others provide opportunities to achieve a hospital presence throughout the service area.

In the facility planning process, questions inevitably arise around the size and number of facilities required to achieve the hospital's strategic purposes. Some strategies require—and some strategists prefer—a hub-and-spoke model, with the central hub being the inpatient campus supported by one or more "big boxes" that house multiple practices and ancillary services, and the spokes being "small boxes" housing solo or small group practices located in targeted neighborhoods. Other strategies and strategists support variations on this hub-and-spoke theme.

Regardless of the market variables, planning for health care facilities (hospitals, medical office buildings, ambulatory care centers, surgery centers, individual medical offices, free-standing imaging centers, and so forth) today should begin with a careful review of the primary care market and its needs, wants, and priorities; growth; and evolution. Developing a clear primary care retail analysis and subsequent development of a retail strategy[2] will help ensure that the numbers, sizes, locations, specialty composition, and ancillary services designed into facilities will meet the current and projected market demand.

For example, in a large urban or suburban setting, a hospital located in the more established part of town may choose to place or affiliate with several primary care practices located in neighborhoods up to thirty minutes away, in the faster growing suburbs across town. In support of those practices, a strategist may decide to place a big box facility within a ten- to fifteen-minute drive of those several primary care locations. The big box might include commonly requested specialty physicians as permanent residents, be used as a satellite location, or serve as the location for specialty rotation through a hot suite. The big box may also include ambulatory surgery, extensive imaging services, laboratory, pharmacy, durable medical equipment, and so forth, again, depending on the needs of local referring physicians and their patients.

The Multispecialty Challenge

Given the increased numbers of specialty physicians being employed by hospitals, some strategists are interested in building facilities to support the formation of multispecialty group practices rather than separate single-specialty offices such as those found in many MOBs. Multispecialty group settings are effective and have been so in a variety of settings over several decades. However, many of these organizations have struggled to overcome the negative impact of large, impersonal reception desks, cavernous waiting rooms, and confusing hallways.

Our preference is to locate single-specialty practice settings off shared hallways, despite the likely additional design and construction cost. This approach dramatically improves the practice's ability to manage the patient experience, which ideally may play out as follows: I, the patient, enter the building and approach a nicely designed directory, which takes me to the proper floor and practice suite. There, I am greeted by a receptionist who has a good chance of knowing (or guessing) my name, and she tells me she has been expecting me. I am seated in a self-contained reception area that has been designed and decorated, with me in mind, with magazines and other features that relate to the unique patient population of which I am a part. The receptionist knows what time I arrived and monitors my wait time. The clinical assistant greets me without a megaphone-like shout and assists me to the examination room, which is a short walk from the reception area. The front end of my experience has been managed in a way that not only pleases me but also facilitates the practice's operational flow.

One other important note about multispecialty group settings is the comfort level of current and potential referring physicians to refer their patients. Often, independent physicians will not refer to specialists in multispecialty groups that include primary care practices—especially those located under the same roof. Their fear (usually unfounded) is that the specialists will not return their referred patients; more often, a referred patient will choose the convenience of having all his or her medical services under one roof and switch to an affiliated primary care physician. Although such changes might be the patient's choice, future referrals will be shifted elsewhere.

Equipment—It's Cheap

People are expensive; by comparison, most equipment is cheap. Rather than save money by purchasing just one, large copy machine, forcing receptionists to leave the reception desk to copy an insurance card, place an additional $100 copy machine at the reception desk. Customer service will improve, receptionist productivity will increase, compliance with this revenue cycle best practice will increase, and movement (confusion) behind the front desk will decrease. The same argument may be made for nursing using a lone fax machine to fax referrals. Certainly, the true costs of such decisions in terms of poor service and lost productivity are often difficult to quantify on the income statement, but the difficulties they create are real nonetheless.

Our recommendations to our clients include buying or leasing the equipment best suited to help their physicians, mid-level providers, support staff members, and management do their jobs efficiently and effectively. Spending more money up front to obtain the additional equipment (clinical or business), the helpful software module, the better desk chair, the faster processor, and so forth is not just an investment in equipment; it is *an investment in people*. We strongly urge our clients not to "cost cut" their way to success in a labor-intensive, service business like a medical practice. Such cost cutting simply does not work.

Cheap Furnishings

Furnishings influence the patient experience and the productivity of practice staff members. Striking the balancing between comfort and durability can be a challenge.

Make the extra investment to find and install furnishings that are comfortable (e.g., have a chair delivered to your office and spend a day sitting in it before you buy), practical (e.g., easily sanitized, with firm armchairs for geriatric offices so patients can get in and out), and durable (e.g., stain resistant for adults, bulletproof and easily replaced for pediatric offices).

Importantly, people tend to prefer to wait in a seat of their own rather than sit on a couch. A reception room should be inviting and warm, but it is not a living room. Lighting and end tables are usually a nice touch, especially if the magazines are current and kept neatly displayed by the receptionist.

Facility Maintenance

A new coat of paint, new carpet, live plants, clean hallways, landscaping, and a striped parking lot are signs of high-quality medical care—at least to those of us who cannot spell some of the services physicians provide to us. Yet patients often encounter threadbare carpet, stained furniture, marked walls, dusty plastic plants, cluttered hallways, dirty elevators, weedy grass, dead bushes, cracked parking lots, and other signs of inattention. We recommend that senior management follow the path of patients entering their facilities rather than parking in the staff lot and entering through a back door. Walk up to the reception desk and see if internal signage and the new patient packet are professional and reasonable in appearance and function. Sit in the reception area and watch and listen. Wander past the examination rooms. Look at the nurses' station. Ask yourself: "If these sights are surrogate measures of our quality care and caring, what message are we communicating?"

Three key challenges face medical practice networks trying to maintain an appropriate appearance. First, many are losing money. They have difficulty convincing decision makers to replace the carpet when precious capital is already being used to stanch operating losses. Second, these facilities are frequently "out of sight and out of mind" for senior management, unless the hospital chief executive officer (CEO) is a market manager visiting primary care and specialty locations. Third, it is often unclear who is responsible for maintaining the hospital-owned practice facility.

We recommend that network management conduct an annual, detailed facilities inventory, supported by digital photos inside and outside. Table 11-1 is a rating scale we use to score facilities and equipment as part of this annual review. It helps create a comparative view of the facilities owned by or leased for the physician network.

We also recommend that the market manager visit every hospital-owned facility at least annually to see what image ambulatory locations are creating for the hospital. Nothing serves to enlist the support of CEOs who care about the image of facilities bearing the hospital's logo like a road trip.

We suggest that practice managers be held accountable for the facilities and equipment in their locations. Managers should work with their practice operations councils to ensure that the annual capital budget includes routine maintenance and upgrades for the facilities and equipment. These capital requests should be prioritized and supported with reliable cost estimates, photos, and other documentation. Importantly, if managers cannot get the attention of hospital maintenance departments, we recommend that they deal with issues and obtain forgiveness later.

Table 11-1. Facilities and Equipment Rating Scale

Rating Scale 1 2 3 4 5 Poor Excellent	Example: Central City Clinic	Write the Clinic Name Below														
Facility location	1															
Parking lot size	3															
Parking lot appearance	5															
Office accessibility from parking	2															
Building exterior	3															
Building grounds	3															
Office furnishings	4															
Office decor	4															
Office floor coverings	4															
Office wall coverings	2															
Office window coverings	2															
Medical equipment	3															
Medical furnishings	4															
Office/business equipment	5															
Office layout/patient flow	3															
Office neatness (absence of clutter)	4															
Office cleanliness	3															
Internal/external signage	2															

Summary

Facilities decisions should be based on the needs, wants, and priorities of the neighborhoods they are intended to serve. Market share is captured in well-placed primary care practices and referred to specialists and to ancillary services conveniently located for that relatively smaller number of patients who require those services. Every medical practice in the network, which sees dozens of patients a week, should look just as nice as the hospital entryway and reception area. "Nice" does not mean $30 per square foot. Rather, it means conveniently located, nicely appointed, comfortably furnished, well equipped, clean, and tidy.

Managers should remember that people are more expensive, and certainly more valuable, than furnishings and equipment. Make sure they have what they need to perform their tasks comfortably, efficiently, and effectively. Poor facilities and equipment are at best a distraction and at worst a detriment to providing high-quality clinical care and a high-quality patient experience.

References

1. M. Halley and A. Little, "Net One, Net Two: The Primary Care Network Income Statement," *Healthcare Financial Management* October (1999): 61–63.
2. M. Halley, *The Primary Care–Market Share Connection: How Hospitals Achieve Competitive Advantage,* 97–111 (Chicago: Health Administration Press, 2007).

CHAPTER 12

Finance and Accounting

Experienced, astute managers have long known that employees improve what managers measure. They also know that performance measurement is a tool that must be used judiciously. Focus staff members on too many outcome indicators (a common challenge in today's computerized world), and the result is beautiful, multicolored dashboards that management hardly has time to update between meetings—let alone effect change based on them. Focus on too few indicators, and their related objectives may be all that are accomplished.

Targeting Key Behaviors

Measuring *for* performance requires a clear understanding of the key behaviors required to achieve our desired outcomes. The performance measures selected must motivate those key behaviors, with the understanding that any other metrics (even if available at the push of a button) are superfluous at best and a distraction at worst.

The authors of the book *Influencer* remind us that the outcomes we seek are a function of what we *do*. Therefore, identifying and measuring what the authors call "vital behaviors" is critical to both short- and long-term success.[1] If we want to measure *for* performance, we must work through the clutter of myriad potential measures to find those vital indicators that both *measure* and *motivate* the key behaviors. Reams of reports, colorful graphs and charts, PowerPoint presentations, and budget variance reports are standard fare in many organizations. Unfortunately, too often these tools camouflage an entity's failure to deliver the desired outcome. Managers become "storytellers" rather than change agents, coming up with a better story each month to justify missed targets. While reporting outcomes is important, measuring for performance requires a focus on behavior—individual behavior.

Engaging individuals in (1) isolating vital behaviors, (2) identifying performance measures, and (3) establishing performance targets is imperative if managers want to achieve peak performance. Fist-pounding bullies do get some results from their threatened employees; even some knowledge workers cower. These same Neanderthal managers then wonder why performance is not sustainable when they are not in the room. Imposing unrealistic budget mandates, an all too common dance in the hospital and health system world of finance, has the same effect, doing little to engage intelligent people in solving real problems by changing their behavior. The resulting "plastic" budgets are owned by the finance department, and management brushes up on its storytelling skills.

Measuring for performance requires the engagement of knowledge workers, support staff, and management, who jointly own the challenges and jointly develop the solutions. Only then will "we" become accountable for bottom-line performance. Finance and accounting professionals support these efforts by accurately identifying the performance constraints, providing historical perspective, teaching about the cost structure, sharing potential tactics, and helping document the impact of implemented strategies. Because all involved understand the strategies and why they must be implemented, they are more likely to change their individual behavior to accommodate their solutions. Couple these tactics with the right performance measures and a frequent opportunity to personally report results, and the organization has a proven recipe for consistent performance improvement and sustainable achievement.

This chapter first reviews the traditional and not-so-traditional measures of outcomes. It then identifies and discusses the implementation of performance-changing behaviors.

How We Measure—It Counts!

On more than one occasion we have listened to previously independent physicians lament that when they owned their practices they were not losing money. They understood what it took to meet a biweekly payroll and to pay the other bills. They understood what it took to produce their own compensation. Now they express frustration over their inability to understand the monthly financial information they receive, let alone to help management solve practice problems. Engaging these experienced physicians in the success of individual practices and the practice network boosts performance improvement.

Perhaps even more challenging are those physicians who have never had to meet a payroll. They have no perspective on and perhaps little interest in the challenges of financial performance. A few years ago our team wrote a book targeted at new physicians leaving residency or fellowship training programs. We were asked why we wrote *The Medical Practice Start-Up Guide* when so many physicians want nothing to do with the business side of medicine.[2] In fact, most want to be employed so that someone else can manage the business and leave them to do what they were trained to do: practice medicine.

Our response is simple. The day physicians leave their training programs, they are in business. Like it or not, the practice of medicine does not occur without revenues and expenses, coding and billing, support staff, and so forth. Whether physicians are employed or independent, business decisions must be made that affect their ability to provide high-quality clinical care in a caring environment. They do themselves and their employers a favor by being willing and able to participate in those decisions rather than grousing about them after they have been made by others.

Employed physicians constantly express concern to us about performance measurement. Some of this concern, of course, is deflecting poor performance. In many cases, however, employed physicians are not even aware of how their practices perform. They are not certain about their personal performance or its impact on the practice. Some question the accuracy of numbers they do not understand based on information they do not trust.

Practice managers are often frustrated by the fact that they cannot explain to their physicians the financial information they receive. Consequently, they may avoid the task. Many previously independent small group practice managers rarely saw the financial statements provided to their physician practice owners. They reconciled their bank statement monthly and confidently wrote checks based on that account balance. Now they are expected to understand unfamiliar general ledger categories, corporate allocations, and this thing called "a cruel accounting."

One does not need an MBA to succeed as a physician or as a practice manager. However, *every* physician and *every* practice manager needs a basic understanding of finance and accounting principles in order to contribute meaningfully to the success of a medical practice. That understanding starts with an accounting model that makes sense for the practice.

We propose a reporting model that separates the traditional small group practice revenue and expenses from what we call "network overhead."[3] The model, introduced in the previous chapter, has two net income lines: net one and net two. While all the numbers still appear on the income statement (no smoke and mirrors allowed), net one includes all those revenues and only those expenses normally found in private practice settings. Net two includes network overhead such as a network executive, corporate allocations, empty office space, and so forth. The accountability implications of net one and net two are compelling when engaging physicians and senior leadership, as illustrated in the following paragraphs.

If defined properly, net one allows physicians and managers to properly compare their financial performance with the gold standard: private practice. Net one revenue categories are those normally found in small group private practices of the same specialty in the community, including ancillary services revenues. If the physician network uses accrual accounting (which we recommend), the rules for estimating net revenues are practice based, using historical contractual write-offs, and are shared openly with the physicians. Expense categories include provider costs, the office manager, support staff members, billing expenses, clinical supplies, malpractice insurance premiums, building occupancy expense (at the actual rates), bad debt, and other private practice expenses. The resulting net income line (net one) is comparable with other practices in the area and should be at breakeven or better.

The space between net one and net two includes the costs of running a physician network, the aforementioned network overhead. Network overhead includes the executive, a physician recruiter, and other team members charged with the responsibility of running the network. It also includes hourly stipends for physicians participating in the network operations council (NOC) and the costs of strategic decisions such as empty space, which allows for future growth.

For example, if strategists choose to open a new four-physician practice in a new neighborhood, starting with one family physician and leaving the rest of the space vacant, the fledgling practice is allocated 25 percent of the office space (or whatever the portion used) in net one and 75 percent (legitimately empty space) is allocated to net two. (We do not recommend any discounting of the cost per square foot, even if it is a poorly negotiated lease.) Finally, net two may include corporate allocations legitimately spread across all system entities but not normally found in private practice settings. Remember, private practices are very conservative in their use of consultants, attorneys, and even accountants, so those system allocations should be tempered.

Holding physicians and managers accountable for net one legitimizes the outcomes tracking process. Net one is a reflection of practice operations comparable to industry benchmarks—especially if the accounting department uses industry standard general ledger definitions provided by the Medical Group Management Association (MGMA) or the American Medical Group Association (AMGA). When physicians and managers feel that they are consistently receiving and understanding legitimate outcomes feedback, they are far more likely to engage in performance management at the practice and individual levels.

Importantly, some health systems have adopted standard general ledger definitions and a net one–net two model across their member organizations in order to improve comparability of their physician employment strategies across markets. This initiative can be a herculean effort but is well worth the trouble in terms of assigning accountability for performance and identifying best performing networks/practices and best practices.

As a point of reference, we offer table 12-1 as a best practice income statement model we have used successfully for several years and slightly modified for a variety of settings.

From Gap to Glory

Accurately reporting outcomes is critical to success in any venture, and especially in a medical practice where margins are thin at best. Properly analyzing those outcomes to determine the reasons for achievement, or lack thereof, is equally essential. Poor analysis has been the cause of much frustration and wasted resource (e.g., time, energy, money) in hospital-owned medical practices, yielding the equivalent of "wild goose chases" in efforts to improve performance.

Table 12-1. Best Practice Income Statement Model

	1	2	3	4	5	6	7	8	9	10
									Fav/(UnFav)	
	Current_MTD	% of Gross Pat. Revenue	Monthly Average	Current_YTD	% of Gross Pat. Revenue	Budget_MTD	Budget_YTD	Prior_YTD	MTD	YTD
REVENUES										
Gross FFS Patient Revenue	146,208	100.00%	146,208	1,754,500	100.00%	150,595	1,807,135	1,579,050	(4.386)	(52,635)
Gross Ancillary Revenue	0	0.00%	0	0	0.00%	0	0	0	0	0
Less Allowance	(43,308)	(29.62%)	(43,308)	(519,695)	(29.62%)	(44,607)	(535,286)	(467,726)	1,299	15,591
Charity Allowance	0	0.00%	0	0	0.00%	0	0	0	0	0
Net Fee-for-Service Revenue	102,900	70.38%	102,900	1,234,805	70.38%	105,987	1,271,849	1,111,325	(3,087)	(37,044)
		% Cap Revenue			**% Cap Revenue**					
Managed Care Per Member Per Month	0	0.00%	0	0	0.00%	0	0	0	0	0
Total Net Revenue	102,900	70.38%	102,900	1,234,805	70.38%	105,987	1,271,849	1,111,325	(3,087)	(37,044)
		% of Tot. Net Rev.			**% of Tot. Net Rev.**					
EXPENSES										
Physician Compensation & Benefits	**49,392**	**48.00%**	**49,392**	**592,706**	**48.00%**	**48,404**	**580,852**	**557,144**	**(988)**	**(11,854)**
Mid-level Compensation & Benefits	**0**	**0.00%**	**0**	**0**	**0.00%**	**0**	**0**	**0**	**0**	**0**
Staff Compensation & Benefits	**32,928**	**32.00%**	**32,928**	**395,138**	**32.00%**	**32,270**	**387,235**	**371,429**	**(659)**	**(7,903)**
Total Employment Expense	82,320	80.00%	82,320	987,844	80.00%	80,674	968,087	928,573	(1,646)	(19,757)
Building Occupancy	**10,290**	**10.00%**	**10,290**	**123,481**	**10.00%**	**10,084**	**121,011**	**116,072**	**(206)**	**(2,470)**
Expendable Clinical Supplies	**8,232**	**8.00%**	**8,232**	**98,784**	**8.00%**	**8,067**	**96,809**	**92,857**	**(165)**	**(1,976)**
Purchased Services	5,145	5.00%	5,145	61,740	5.00%	5,042	60,505	58,036	(103)	(1,235)
Purchased Services Ancillary Expense	0	0.00%	0	0	0.00%	0	0	0	0	0
Purchased Services—Other	0	0.00%	0	0	0.00%	0	0	0	0	0
Ancillary Expense Adjustment	0	0.00%	0	0	0.00%	0	0	0	0	0
Equipment	2,200	2.14%	2,200	26,400	2.14%	2,156	25,872	24,816	(44)	(528)
Telephone	1,200	1.17%	1,200	14,400	1.17%	1,176	14,112	13,536	(24)	(288)
Other Supplies	900	0.87%	900	10,800	0.87%	882	10,584	10,152	(18)	(216)
Insurance	3,000	2.92%	3,000	36,000	2.92%	2,940	35,280	33,840	(60)	(720)
Other Expenses	4,000	3.89%	4,000	48,000	3.89%	3,920	47,040	45,120	(80)	(960)
Bad Debts	750	0.73%	750	9,000	0.73%	735	8,820	8,460	(15)	(180)
Total Expenses	118,037	114.71%	118,037	1,416,449	114.71%	115,677	1,388,120	1,331,462	(2,361)	(28,329)
Income (Loss) from Operations	(15,137)	(14.71%)	(15,137)	(181,644)	(14.71%)	(9,689)	(116,271)	(220,138)	(5,448)	(65,373)
Excess Building Capacity	0	0.00%	0	0	0.00%	0	0	0	0	0
Other Net Two Revenue	0	0.00%	0	0	0.00%	0	0	0	0	0
Other Net Two Expense	0	0.00%	0	0	0.00%	0	0	0	0	0
Ancillary Reversal from Net One	0	0.00%	0	0	0.00%	0	0	0	0	0
Corporate Allocation	(5,000)	(4.86%)	(5,000)	(60,000)	(4.86%)	(3,500)	(48,000)	(52,000)	(1,500)	(12,000)
Management Fees	(500)	(0.49%)	(500)	(6,000)	(0.49%)	(750)	(1,000)	(12,000)	250	(5,000)
Goodwill/Non-compete Amortization	0	0.00%	0	0	0.00%	0	0	0	0	0
Interest Income	0	0.00%	0	0	0.00%	0	0	0	0	0
Net Income (Loss)	(20,637)	(20.06%)	(20,637)	(247,644)	(20.06%)	(13,939)	(165,271)	(284,138)	(6,698)	(82,373)

Note: FFS = fee-for-service; MTD = month to date; YTD = year to date. Totals subject to rounding error.

Monthly Variances

Proper evaluation of medical practice performance is a multidimensional exercise. Using table 12-1, we first compare current month-to-date performance with the monthly average outcomes (columns 1 and 3, respectively). A practice manager's ability to first understand and then explain variances in outcomes from the current month compared with the monthly average is an essential starting point. This exercise raises issues about recent contributing factors and/or misallocated expenses and helps the manager understand the impact of operating decisions, including performance improvement tactics.

Ratio Analysis

The second most important performance measurement dimension involves ratio analysis. Standard balance sheet financial ratios do not apply in the medical practice business. The most meaningful ratios are those comparing revenue and expense categories with the net revenue (accrual) or collections (cash basis) line of the income statement. (Both MGMA and AMGA provide comparative results across numerous revenue and expense ratios.) Comparing current month ratios with year-to-date ratios (table 12-1, columns 2 and 5, respectively) is another powerful analytical exercise. The labor-intensive nature of the medical practice business allows few scale economies. This fact becomes more pronounced as practices reach their current productive capacity. Increased volume results in increased physician compensation, higher support staff expenses (often including overtime), and increased clinical supply costs. If viewed in isolation, an increase in support staff costs might be cause for alarm. But if viewed as a percentage of additional net patient revenue, support staff costs may actually be lower than in prior periods.

In the hospital business, standard indicators of performance across the industry include the number of full-time-equivalent (FTE) employees assigned to a particular task. The number of FTE support staff per physician is often applied to physician offices as the benchmark indicator. While this ratio can be useful, it is not the most effective measure of support staff, as physician productivity often varies widely even within the same group practice. The best measure of productive capacity and efficiency is the staff cost ratio, which is support staff costs divided by net patient revenue. Medical practice industry experts have long known that busier physicians always require more support staff (FTEs) than their less productive counterparts do. Their additional net patient revenue, however, usually more than offsets the cost of additional staff. In other words, the staff cost ratio is actually lower.

Best practice outcomes performance reporting includes ratios in three categories: several *financial* ratios, several *workload* ratios and statistics, and the standard *employment* ratios that include FTE calculations per provider. These ratios are viewed for current month data and compared with year-to-date performance and an external benchmark.

Common financial ratios include the following:

- Provider cost ratio (provider costs/net patient revenue)
- Staff cost ratio (support staff costs/net patient revenue)
- Building occupancy ratio (all facilities costs/net patient revenue)
- Clinical supply cost ratio (clinical supplies/net patient revenue)
- Purchased services cost ratio (purchased services/net patient revenue)
- Total nonprovider cost ratio (total nonprovider costs/net patient revenue)
- Gross revenue per provider (gross revenue/provider FTE)
- Total net revenue per provider (net revenue/provider FTE)
- Gross patient revenue per visit (gross patient revenue/total ambulatory visits)
- Total net revenue per visit (net patient revenue/total ambulatory visits)

For the purposes of defining provider FTEs, we usually count a mid-level provider as 50 percent of an FTE physician, based on our experience with mid-level charges and productivity.

Our common workload ratios include the following:

- New patient visits
- New patient ratio (new patients/total patient visits)
- Ambulatory visits
- Hospital and other visits
- Total visits
- Work relative value units (wRVUs)
- Coding index (wRVUs/total visits)

Gap Analysis

Although ratio analysis is an extremely valuable tool, the obvious challenge of using net revenue as the denominator for many of these ratios is the number of factors that can negatively affect net revenue. Inadequate gross charges (e.g., a new practice), a poor payer mix, and a flawed revenue cycle can invalidate traditional efforts at ratio analysis. Our gap analysis process (table 12-2) adjusts for this challenge.

The term *gap analysis* is not unique to medical practice analysis. Our approach, however, is unique and makes use of standard medical ratios and benchmark data for financially viable practices. We start with dollar figures taken directly from five categories in the practice income statement. Column 1 of table 12-2 highlights the year-to-date practice loss and the five categories. Column 2 illustrates the income statement results. Column 3 incorporates ratios for sustainable practice

Table 12-2. Gap Analysis

1	2	3	4	5	6	7
YTD Loss ($120,435)	Actual	Sustainable Ratios	Sustainable Dollars	Difference to Actual	Sustainable Benchmark Net Revenue	Difference to Actual
Net revenue	$1,234,805				$1,612,500	$377,695
Provider cost	$595,706	.41	$508,678	($84,029)	$664,269	$71,563
Staff cost	$395,138	.26	$319,024	($76,113)	$416,606	$21,468
Building occupancy	$123,481	.07	$83,238	($40,242)	$108,699	($14,782)
Clinical supplies	$55,584	.04	$50,133	($5,451)	$65,468	$9,884

Note: YTD = year to date.

performance. Often those ratios are MGMA or AMGA medians for the specialty. Column 4 is derived by multiplying actual net revenue ($1,234,805) by the ratio in each of the four expense categories. Column 4 is the amount we can afford to pay at the actual net revenue. Column 5 illustrates the difference between the actual dollars spent and what is sustainable in each category at the current net revenue. Column 6 identifies the expected net revenue for the number of FTE physicians and mid-level providers (at 50 percent of an FTE physician) serving in the practice. (We usually recommend the 60th percentile net revenue figures for the specialty, which in this case yields expected net revenue of $1,612,500.) If the sustainable benchmark net revenue is less than the actual net patient revenue, use columns 1–5 for your gap analysis. If actual net revenue is short, complete columns 6 and 7. Column 6 also illustrates the costs that could be incurred under the sustainable benchmark net revenue by multiplying the $1,612,500 by the sustainable ratios in column 3. Column 7 compares the actual dollars spent (column 2) with the potential dollars in column 6.

In this case, the practice is losing $120,435 (column 1). If we only use the income statement ratios (columns 1–5), we might assume that expense controls need to be imposed to solve the problem. The real problem, however, is revenue. Cutting expenses will often only exacerbate the performance problem by reducing productivity. If we find a way to drive volume and revenue, most of the expense issues resolve themselves, as does the majority of the loss.

Budget Comparisons

The third slice of performance comparison is the common budget comparison. Some years, comparisons to budget are a useful third cut at the data. Other years, budget comparisons are an exercise in futility. Most budgets are static. Most organizations do not spend the time and energy to maintain variable budgets. (Some organizational leaders are afraid of losing any level of accountability if they employ variable budgeting.) Our budgets are developed months in advance using historical data and our best guess about how the practice and the environment will change between budget submission and the beginning of the fiscal year.

Most crystal balls are cloudy, at best. Any significant change can render a static budget useless. Losing one of the four physicians in a practice right after the fiscal year begins means the loss of 25 percent or more of productive capacity. Some expenses can, and will, be reduced, but explaining hard-dollar variances is a waste of time and energy. A failed physician recruitment effort has a similar effect on a static budget. Still, barring these types of significant change, budget comparisons can provide a useful look at performance against the desired outcome.

The Site-Specific Action Plan

While a variety of network-wide initiatives facilitate or become barriers to practice performance, medical practice networks achieve financial viability one practice, even one physician, at a time. Without practice-specific focus and accountability, there is no financial viability.

In properly functioning networks, practice operations councils (POCs) are charged with achieving break-even or better performance at net one, with their practice managers providing the implementation support. The rigor necessary to meet this challenge is a function of monthly attention to two critical documents: the income statement, which documents current and comparative outcomes, and the site-specific action plan (SSAP), which documents the process-changing and behavior-changing revenue and expense tactics that will yield the desired outcome.

Tactics are developed or discussed in the POC meeting. They are documented on the SSAP along with the estimated financial impact of each. Each tactic is also assigned a responsible party to drive its implementation. The responsible party and the POC determine a timeline for completion, and implementation begins. Each month, the POC reviews the SSAP and holds responsible parties accountable for implementation progress. Practice operations council members also hold each other accountable for sponsorship of the initiatives. Pet projects or people (e.g., "Not my nurse") are not allowed to stymie progress.

On a monthly basis the income statement is carefully reviewed for evidence of tactical implementation. If the SSAP called for a $1,500 improvement, POC members look for that improvement on the revenue or expense side, as appropriate. If that evidence is not found, additional tactics are employed until the evidence of performance improvement becomes overwhelming. Over time, losses are replaced by gains, and the POC can celebrate its achievement with the practice manager and support staff members.

A variety of revenue and expense tactics have been employed by successful POCs over the years, including the following:

- *Physicians per square foot.* One group of doctors realized that their primary care office space was too expensive. Saddled with a long-term lease, they decided to increase the use of the space by adding more providers per square foot. Rather than adopt the traditional 9:00 AM to 5:00 PM appointment model, they decided to supplement their after-hours walk-in clinic with an appointment track. They took turns participating in an 8:00 AM to 2:00 PM/2:00 PM to 8:00 PM appointment track, which allowed two physicians to see a full slate of patients using the same set of examination rooms twelve hours each day. One physician took the early shift, and the other took the late shift. Because the evening shifts were shared, no single physician had an unfair burden and the mid-level provider staffing the extended-hours walk-in practice had easy access to a physician, who was in the building seeing patients by appointment. More providers could be accommodated, and the negative impact of high rent became moot.
- *Appointment schedule.* It is common for physicians to voluntarily change their appointment schedules, adding a few additional morning visits or committing to show up on time. Most practices quickly realize that having someone see patients through the lunch hour can be a real boon, adding patients to the practice each day. Patients, of course, are pleased to have more convenient hours available.
- *Overtime.* A common target for POCs is overtime. Why pay time-and-a-half for straight-time work? By working together, physicians and managers can reduce or eliminate most overtime (allowing for the unexpected, on occasion). Sometimes POCs choose to add full-time or part-time staff to eliminate persistent overtime.
- *Highest and best-use staffing.* Giving clinical assistants permission to manage physician productivity is increasingly common in highly productive practices. That permission and the training/scripting that follows ensure that the physician's schedule can accommodate a few more patients every day.
- *Chart hunt.* One group of physicians worked with their medical records clerks and their clinical assistants to change the way paper charts moved around the office. They reduced the chart hunt from fourteen potential locations to seven. They also required physicians and nurses to turn around the charts more quickly and the medical records department to file all loose forms and charts within twenty-four hours. The results were nothing short of amazing. The 4-foot stack of loose forms was soon eliminated. Frustration over "missing" documentation declined

dramatically. While not totally eliminated, the number of lost charts dropped by more than half, as did the time required to locate a missing chart.

These and hundreds of other effective tactics are developed and sponsored by POCs and their practice managers every year. Processes are changed, behaviors are modified, commitments are made and kept, failures are identified and overcome, and successes are celebrated.

Obviously, the need for accurate, timely, relevant, and trusted financial reporting (particularly income statements) is critical to the success of this site-specific endeavor. In addition to using those reporting mechanisms, POCs can assess their progress each month by recording revenue and expense tactics and highlighting the income statement outcomes in the SSAP format provided in Appendix B.

A Legitimate Budgeting Process

Despite the challenges of static operating budgets, they are still helpful baselines against which to compare actual experience. The key to successful budgeting in a medical practice network (and in any other setting) is aligning *accountability* for performance with *ownership* of the budget. Ownership is a function of involvement in setting performance targets and developing tactics to achieve those targets. Senior leaders or financial officers must take special care to keep physicians and practice managers involved in establishing targets and tactics or risk disengaging them from the budget. A legitimate budgeting process keeps them engaged through the following actions:

1. Providing a clear budgeting process and a timeline adequate to involve physicians in completing the process
2. Understanding the practice revenue structure and documenting anticipated changes to that structure, including the following:
   a. Engaging physicians and mid-level providers in estimating volume and growth rates based on historical data
   b. Documenting the impact of new services
   c. Estimating the impact of additional provider capacity
   d. Identifying opportunities for coding improvement
   e. Documenting the net effect of pricing changes
   f. Estimating reimbursement changes (contracts and payer mix)
3. Understanding the medical practice cost structure, including:
   a. Fixed, variable, step variable costs
   b. Ratio analysis to anticipate changes as volume changes
   c. Anticipated cost increases

4. Applying ratios with POCs to test preliminary budgets against targets
5. Identifying barriers to reaching targeted performance
6. Engaging POCs in establishing their own stretch goals to reach targets
7. Documenting revenue and expense tactics in an SSAP to demonstrate how targets will be reached
8. Submitting budget and SSAP for final approval
9. Monitoring performance and changing circumstances
10. Adjusting SSAP tactics to achieve performance
11. Monitoring performance

Honoring this participative process allows physicians and managers to struggle with performance realities and, in response, develop tactics to achieve the desired outcome. As long as those outcomes are realistic and the physicians own the tactics, they own the budget. Unrealistic outcomes/expectations or arbitrarily imposed tactics shift ownership of the resulting budget away from the physicians and practice managers, who are in the best position to help ensure successful implementation.

Similarly, capital budgeting starts at the POC with capital requests being prioritized by that group. Financial experts assist each POC in justifying capital budget requests using the four critical success filters: clinical quality, service quality, physician productivity, and operational and financial viability. Usually, capital requests are further prioritized and approved by the NOC before being forwarded to the hospital board for final approval. When capital is allocated, the NOC facilitates its distribution among the POCs.

Summary

Measuring for performance engages every physician and other provider at every practice in the pursuit of realistic performance targets. The right measures focus POCs and their managers on those vital behaviors that will ensure operational and financial success, which is usually defined as the private practice gold standard.

Finance experts understand that the performance measures for medical practice networks differ from those used in hospital settings. They also understand that owning a network produces costs not normally found in private practice settings, and they are careful not to commingle network overhead with site-specific costs. They ensure that physicians are able to properly interpret timely and trustworthy financial information using appropriate ratios that can be compared with relevant industry benchmarks. Physicians are held accountable for legitimate budget targets, which they own, and POCs help design the tactics to achieve those targets, which are recorded in a site-specific action plan. Importantly, performance measures are viewed as helpful tools rather than as oppressive weapons.

References

1. K. Patterson, J. Grenny, D. Maxfield, and R. McMillan, *Influencer: The Power to Change Anything,* 43 (New York: McGraw-Hill, 2007).
2. M. Halley and M. Ferry, *The Medical Practice Start-Up Guide* (Phoenix, MD: Greenbranch, 2008).
3. M. Halley and A. Little, "Net One, Net Two: The Primary Care Network Income Statement." *Healthcare Financial Management* October (1999): 61–63.

Epilogue

The definition of insanity frequently attributed to Albert Einstein is "doing the same thing over and over again and expecting different results." Here we are again—hospital executives employing physicians and making many of the same mistakes their predecessors made between 1985 and 1998. Not surprisingly, we are getting the same results.

Fortunately, we have the opportunity to learn from past mistakes by applying the correct principles identified in this book. Every market is unique, competitive strategies differ, and legal models vary in response to state law. But the basic principles for operating successful individual medical practices are the same from one end of the United States to the other; so, too, are the fundamentals of operating a successful *network* of practices the same from coast to coast.

We have provided consulting and interim management services to hospital clients in more than sixty cities in the past four years. Those that have adopted correct operating principles have made progress. Those that have not done so, perhaps due to contractual constraints, poor planning, fear of change, or just plain arrogance, have not fared so well.

Physician-hospital integration is, once again, "all the rage." It is critical today that chief executive officer (CEO)–market managers base their integration initiatives on a very clear competitive strategy. That strategy must address four business imperatives: (1) capture and control market share, (2) demonstrate clinical and service quality, (3) create capital for reinvestment, and (4) ensure high physician productivity.[1]

Physician employment has the potential to be a viable and sustainable integration tactic if its implementation is based on correct principles. We recommend that every new or established hospital-owned network pause to consider and develop an operating plan that documents physician and executive leaders' understanding of and commitment to best practices in the areas of operational governance, management infrastructure, network development, practice and network marketing, human resource management, practice operations, revenue cycle management, information technology, facilities and equipment, and finance and accounting. Doing so will help ensure commitment to correct principles when the inevitable expediencies surface.

Recognizing that hospital board members are frequently being asked to support hospital ownership of medical practices, we suggest that board members ask their CEO and physician leaders the following questions:[2]

- What is our plan for capturing market share in primary care practices located in critical neighborhoods throughout our service area?
- How are we engaging employed physician leaders as partners in our hospital-owned physician network?
- Are some members of our team experienced in managing financially and operationally viable hospital-owned medical practice networks?
- How are we monitoring clinical quality and service quality within our hospital-owned medical practice network?
- Do our employed physicians understand that break-even financial performance is the minimum performance standard for our established practices and physicians?
- Are we closely monitoring our investment practices (those with new physicians) to make sure they achieve the break-even standard within twenty-four months?

The success of hospital-owned medical practice networks depends on a successful partnership between physician leaders and the hospital CEO (the board-appointed fiduciary). That partnership shares a clear and compelling vision for their integrated future. Implementation is based on correct operating principles for successful medical practices in support of the capital-generating engine. The resulting capital is not wasted on practice operating losses. Rather, the CEO reinvests that capital in strategic primary care and specialty practices and hospital service lines to meet the needs of the communities served. Such integrated partnerships ensure their own sustainability in the years ahead, despite the inevitable challenges.

References

1. M. Halley, "Four Business Imperatives to Manage Dynamic Change in the New Healthcare Environment," *MGMA Connexion* July (2010): 51–54.
2. M. Halley, "Here We Go Again," *Trustee* 63, no. 2 (2010): 12–16.

APPENDIX A

Role Description for the Network Operations Council Chairperson

Origination date: 02/2010 **Revision date:** 04/2010

FLSA status: Exempt **Reports to:** Hospital CEO

GENERAL DESCRIPTION

The network operations council chairperson is accountable to the hospital CEO to facilitate the successful implementation of the network operations council (NOC) model. The chairperson ensures that the NOC efficiently and effectively handles its business during monthly council meetings, which the chairperson facilitates. The chairperson also assists the hospital CEO in managing behavioral and clinical challenges among employed physicians.

PRIMARY DUTIES AND RESPONSIBILITIES

1. Sets a personal example of the four critical success filters: clinical quality, service quality, personal productivity, and practice viability
2. Is a member of and chairs the monthly NOC meetings; in conjunction with the hospital CEO and with the assistance of the network executive, develops the monthly NOC agenda
3. Facilitates NOC strategy and policy discussions; ensures that NOC meeting discussions comply with the basic tenets established by the council; understands the principles of dialogue and ensures their implementation in all NOC and subcommittee meetings[1]
4. Assigns physician chairpersons to NOC subcommittees and communicates with them to make sure those committees fulfill their charters; is an ex officio member of all subcommittees and attends committee meetings as needed
5. Regularly consults with the network executive to provide both clinical and business perspectives on implementation issues in the practice sites; receives reports on implementation progress from the network executive
6. Participates with the hospital CEO in resolving employed-physician behavioral and clinical issues; provides both clinical and practice operations perspectives to the hospital CEO, who is accountable for signing physician employment contracts

POSITION REQUIREMENTS

1. Skills and Abilities

Demonstrated ability to effectively communicate both verbally and in writing; demonstrated comfort with participating in both strategic and tactical discussions; understanding of the business and clinical sides of medicine

2. Education

MD or DO

3. Experience

Excellent leadership track record in a group practice or network setting; hospital or medical staff leadership experience and private practice experience preferred

4. Physical Demands

Will spend time communicating with others by phone and in person; will have some early morning and evening meetings outside of practice hours; will be expected to fulfill a time commitment of 12–15 hours per month in addition to clinical practice hours

---

Note: FLSA = Fair Labor Standards Act.

1. P. Senge, *The Fifth Discipline,* 238–249 (New York: Doubleday, 1990).

APPENDIX B

Site-Specific Action Plan

Site: ______________________________

Manager: ___________________________

Date: ______________________________

Source: The Halley Consulting Group, LLC (www.halleyconsulting.com), copyright © 2006. Reprinted with permission.

Practice Financial Realities

Enter the appropriate net one income/loss from the practice financial statements on a monthly basis

Monthly Average—Net One Income/Loss											
September	October	November	December	January	February	March	April	May	June	July	August
Current Month—Net One Income/Loss											
September	October	November	December	January	February	March	April	May	June	July	August
Current Month—Practice Ambulatory Encounters											
September	October	November	December	January	February	March	April	May	June	July	August
Current Month—Practice Work RVUs											
September	October	November	December	January	February	March	April	May	June	July	August

Note: RVU = relative value unit.

Source: The Halley Consulting Group, LLC (www.halleyconsulting.com), copyright © 2006. Reprinted with permission.

Revenue Enhancement Strategies

Tactics	Person Responsible	Projected Completion Date	Actual Completion Date	$ Amount Change

Total Practice Net Revenue

Enter the appropriate net revenue from the practice financial statements on a monthly basis

Monthly Average—Net Revenue											
September	October	November	December	January	February	March	April	May	June	July	August
Current Month—Net Revenue											
September	October	November	December	January	February	March	April	May	June	July	August

Source: The Halley Consulting Group, LLC (www.halleyconsulting.com), copyright © 2006. Reprinted with permission.

Expense Reduction Strategies

Tactics	Person Responsible	Projected Completion Date	Actual Completion Date	$ Amount Change

Total Practice Net One Expense

Enter the appropriate net one expense from the practice financial statements on a monthly basis

Monthly Average—Net One Expense											
September	October	November	December	January	February	March	April	May	June	July	August
Current Month—Net One Expense											
September	October	November	December	January	February	March	April	May	June	July	August

Source: The Halley Consulting Group, LLC (www.halleyconsulting.com), copyright © 2006. Reprinted with permission.

Qualitative Issues and Tactics

Action Area	Person Responsible	Completion Date	Actual Completion Date	Notes/Remarks
Operations				
Retail Readiness and Customer Service				
Human Resources (Provider and Staff)				
Clinical Quality, Regulatory and Compliance				
Information System				
Other				

Source: The Halley Consulting Group, LLC (www.halleyconsulting.com), copyright © 2006. Reprinted with permission.

APPENDIX C

Physician Candidate Questionnaire

[Physician Candidate]

[Date conducted]

Conducted by:
[ ]

Source: The Halley Consulting Group, LLC (www.halleyconsulting.com), copyright © 2008. Reprinted with permission.

Table of Contents

Section 1

Demographic Information

1. Please provide the requested information below:

General Information

Physician Name	Specialty(s)
Email address	**Mailing Address**
Work Telephone	**Home Telephone**
Spouse Name	**Spouse Profession**
Date available to start practice	

Source: The Halley Consulting Group, LLC (www.halleyconsulting.com), copyright © 2008. Reprinted with permission.

Section 2

Education and Training

✔ C.V. Attached

2. Describe any special training and qualifications

3. Describe your most interesting experience

4. Describe your most difficult experience

5. Recommendations for improvement

6. Describe your special accomplishments

Source: The Halley Consulting Group, LLC (www.halleyconsulting.com), copyright © 2008. Reprinted with permission.

Section 3

Licenses and Certification

✔ C.V. Attached

Section 4

Practice Experience

Current Practice

7. Major areas of responsibility

8. Time commitment

9. Call coverage

10. Patient volumes/dollars

Source: The Halley Consulting Group, LLC (www.halleyconsulting.com), copyright

11. Staff (Employees)

12. Administration

13. Governance

14. Peers

15. Communication

Source: The Halley Consulting Group, LLC (www.halleyconsulting.com), copyright © 2008. Reprinted with permission.

Previous Practice

16. Major areas of responsibility

17. Time commitment

18. Call coverage

19. Patient volumes/dollars

20. Staff (Employees)

Source: The Halley Consulting Group, LLC (www.halleyconsulting.com), copyright © 2008. Reprinted with permission.

21. Administration

22. Governance

23. Peers

24. Communication

Source: The Halley Consulting Group, LLC (www.halleyconsulting.com), copyright © 2008. Reprinted with permission.

Section 5

Desired Practice Situation

✔ Define Absolutes

25. Type (Single specialty group, solo, office sharing, etc.)

26. Preferred group specialty and specialty composition

27. Preferred call coverage

28. Employee expectations

Source: The Halley Consulting Group, LLC (www.halleyconsulting.com), copyright

29. Inpatient/outpatient/ambulatory mix

30. Patient volume

31. Governance

32. Hospital affiliation

33. Geographic location

Source: The Halley Consulting Group, LLC (www.halleyconsulting.com), copyright © 2008. Reprinted with permission.

34. Physical facility preferences

35. Partners

36. Start-up assistance

37. Special equipment needs (office and hospital)

Source: The Halley Consulting Group, LLC (www.halleyconsulting.com), copyright © 2008. Reprinted with permission.

Section 6

Income and Benefits

38. Desired income for the first and second year

39. Desired financial arrangement (salary, percentage, combination, etc.)

40. Time off (vacation, CME, other)

41. Other benefits (health insurance, disability insurance, dental insurance, retirement)

Section 7

Community Characteristics

42. Size

43. Geographic preference

44. Seasons

45. Cost-of-living

46. Housing

Source: The Halley Consulting Group, LLC (www.halleyconsulting.com), copyright © 2008. Reprinted with permission.

47. Schools

48. Higher education

49. Job market

50. Social activities: How does candidate spend his/her free time?

51. What activities/amenities are important in a desired city/town/practice location?

Source: The Halley Consulting Group, LLC (www.halleyconsulting.com), copyright © 2008. Reprinted with permission.

52. Proximity to family *(candidate indicated this information voluntarily)*

Section 8

Family Interests

Physician

53. What activities outside of work are you interested in?

54. Hobbies

55. Education

56. Sports

Source: The Halley Consulting Group, LLC (www.halleyconsulting.com), copyright © 2008. Reprinted with permission.

57. Leisure activities

Spouse *(information provided by candidate—not asked by interviewer)*

58. Career

59. Cultural activities

60. Hobbies

61. Education

Source: The Halley Consulting Group, LLC (www.halleyconsulting.com), copyright © 2008. Reprinted with permission.

62. Sports

63. Leisure activities

64. Children *(information offered voluntarily by candidate—interviewer did not ask)*

Children

Name	Age	Interests

Source: The Halley Consulting Group, LLC (www.halleyconsulting.com), copyright © 2008. Reprinted with permission.

Section 9

Personal Characteristics

65. Greatest strengths

66. Areas you would like to improve

67. Reason you entered medicine

68. Have your reasons changed?

69. What do you like least about your profession?

---

70. If you had to choose a different career . . .

71. On a scale of 1–10 (with 10 being high), please score each of the following attributes as they relate to your personality:

1 Low	2 3 4 5 6 7 8 9 10 High
	a. Shy
	b. Aggressive
	c. High energy
	d. Sociable
	e. Sense of humor
	f. Able to manage stress
	g. Common sense
	h. Motivation level
	i. Achievement oriented

72. Have you selected some long-term objectives you can share?

73. Have you determined what role money plays in your motivation?

Source: The Halley Consulting Group, LLC (www.halleyconsulting.com), copyright © 2008. Reprinted with permission.

Section 10

Interview Experience

74. How many sites have you or do you plan to visit?

75. When do you expect to make a decision?

76. What kind of packages have you seen your associates offered?

77. What are the key factors that you think will affect your decision?

Source: The Halley Consulting Group, LLC (www.halleyconsulting.com), copyright © 2008. Reprinted with permission.

APPENDIX D

Term Sheet for Initial Offer of Employment

For Discussion Only—Not a Legally Binding Agreement

Topic	Term (sample only)
Term of employment: We recommend an initial term of 24 months for primary care physicians *new* to the area (as little as 12 months for invasive specialists). For *established* physicians, we recommend 1-year "evergreen" contracts with the option for either party to give a 90-day notice to end the contract without cause at any time.	Initial term runs 24 months, from July 1, 20__ through July 31, 20__. Renewal options available annually thereafter. 90-day notice without cause.
Assigned location: Clarifies for the parties the assigned location(s) where the physician will be expected to provide services.	Short North Internal Medicine 7229 Belvedere Ave., Suite 109 Columbus, OH 43017
Physician duties: Identifies a few key duties and performance expectations. Successful (viable) private practice standards become the minimum ante to participate in the network. We usually discuss the fact that productivity has to be consistent with private practice and must yield a viable practice setting. We also discuss the importance of "referring domestic," meaning referring to affiliated specialists and hospital inpatient and outpatient services. This discussion highlights the hospital's role (with the help of specialty physicians) as the capital-generating engine for the integrated system.	Full time. Productivity consistent with private practice. Schedule consistent with private practice. Equal share of call coverage with other providers in the group. Referral management.
Fixed compensation: Identifies that portion of the compensation that is fixed over a given time frame.	A rate of $160,000 annually during the initial term. Salary to be paid biweekly over 26 weeks per year at $6,153.85 per pay period.
Productivity compensation: Identifies the productivity model as well as how and when the physician can and must move to productivity compensation. Established physicians whose practices are acquired are expected to move immediately to the productivity model once they become employed.	Opportunity to shift from fixed compensation to a productivity compensation model at physician's discretion at any time during the initial term. Election to move to productivity model is irrevocable. Productivity compensation required, starting with the first renewal term on August 1, 20__. In discussing the productivity compensation model, we always refer to the rate per work relative value unit as "the rate then in effect for the specialty" rather than placing a specific rate in the contract document.

Topic	Term (sample only)
Employee benefits: Describes the benefits package in general terms and uses attachments for greater detail.	Current physician benefit package (attached).
Allowed time off (ATO): Identifies the ATO limits. Allowed time off is preferable when physicians are on an appropriate productivity compensation approach. Allowed time off has no cash value.	Physician will receive 20 days of vacation time annually at the beginning of the year. Eligible to use vacation after 90 days. Base salary continues. Carryover policies.
Sick leave: Identifies allowed time for sick leave, which looks and acts like ATO but is kept as a separate bank.	Physician will receive 5 days of sick leave annually. Base salary continues. Carryover policies.
Continuing medical education (CME): Identifies the time allowed and the reimbursement for continuing education. Similar to private practice, physicians are allowed time off for CME.	Physician will receive 5 days per calendar year of paid time off for continuing medical education. Physician will be allowed up to $3,000 in expense reimbursement for actual cost of attendance at pre-approved CME, journals, professional memberships, and professional dues. Base salary continues.
Malpractice: Providing malpractice for employment physicians, including tail coverage should they leave the employ of the organization, is a best practice to protect the physician and the organization.	Davis Medical Center (DMC) will provide malpractice coverage effective on physician's first day of employment and will provide tail coverage through the last day of employment if physician leaves DMC employment.
Noncompete: A touchy, but essential, term of any physician employment contract. Represents and protects investment in market share and in referral management.	Time frame is 2 years after employment terminates. Five-mile radius of assigned practice location for primary care physicians. Fifteen-mile radius of assigned practice location for specialty physicians.
Nondiversion: Helps keep the peace should a breakup occur. The effect of contract termination is defined to help protect market share and reset referral patterns.	No direct patient solicitation or employee solicitation upon termination. Mass media advertising and Yellow Pages permitted if location is outside the required noncompete radius.
Nondisclosure: A covenant not to share confidential information with a new employer or others, including the way business is conducted.	Will not reveal corporation's confidential information.

APPENDIX E

Physician Practice Start-Up Action Plan Summary

[Health Care Facility Name]

[Street Address]

[City, ST ZIP Code]

[Phone]

Professional Svcs (Provider) Agmt.	Action	Project Coordinator	Target Date	Start Date	Completion Date	Notes
Professional Services (Provider) Agreement	1. Employment agreement drafted by legal counsel					
	2. Draft employment agreement to senior leadership and/or Board for review and feedback					
	3. Draft employment agreement approved and finalized					
	4. Employment agreement to physician(s)					
	5. Execute employment agreement					
	6. Route and file executed employment agreement to: a. Legal Counsel—original b. Human Resources—copy c. Corporate Administration—copy d. Network—copy e. Physician—copy					

Source: The Halley Consulting Group, LLC (www.halleyconsulting.com), copyright © 2006. Reprinted with permission.

Physician Employment	Action	Project Coordinator	Target Date	Start Date	Completion Date	Notes
Physician Employment	1. Provider employment applications completed					
	2. Benefits explained and forms completed					
	3. Tax withholding forms completed					
	4. Direct deposit authorization					
	5. Employment eligibility verification completed					
	6. Employment physical scheduled					
	7. Copy of curriculum vitae obtained					
	8. Copy of medical license obtained					
	9. Copy of Federal DEA certificate obtained					
	10. Copy of state controlled substance certificate obtained					
	11. Copy of Driver's License and Social Security Card					
	12. Copy of current Malpractice Insurance Coverage/ Proof of Tail Coverage if applicable					

Physician Cred./ Managed Care	Action	Project Coordinator	Target Date	Start Date	Completion Date	Notes
Physician Credentialing/ Managed Care	1. Determine legal entity status and obtain Tax ID number					
	2. Determine payer contracts to be established with managed care plans					
	3. Obtain & complete payer credentialing applications					
	4. Complete Medicare & Medicaid applications					
	5. Complete Clinical Laboratory Improvement Amendments (CLIA) application					

Source: The Halley Consulting Group, LLC (www.halleyconsulting.com), copyright © 2006. Reprinted with permission.

Physician Cred./ Managed Care	Action	Project Coordinator	Target Date	Start Date	Completion Date	Notes
	6. Obtain physician/hospital signatures on applications					
	7. Hand deliver/submit payer contracts to companies					
	8. Apply for Hospital(s) privileges					

Staff Employment	Action	Project Coordinator	Target Date	Start Date	Completion Date	Notes
Staff Employment	1. Identify staff positions					
	2. Develop job descriptions					
	3. Determine salary ranges					
	4. Employee requisitions approved					
	5. Develop training and orientation for employees (Training and Orientation listing attached)					
	6. Job posted/advertised					
	7. Internal applicants interviewed					
	8. External applicants interviewed					
	9. Employment applications completed					
	10. Employment offer(s) extended					
	11. Employment physical completed					
	12. Benefits explained and forms completed					
	13. Background check completed					
	14. Tax withholding forms completed					
	15. Direct deposit authorization obtained					
	16. Training on time clocking procedures					

Source: The Halley Consulting Group, LLC (www.halleyconsulting.com), copyright © 2006. Reprinted with permission.

Facility—Leased	Action	Project Coordinator	Target Date	Start Date	Completion Date	Notes
Facility—Leased	1. Space needs identified (including build out requirements)					
	2. Preferred locations identified					
	3. Financial Feasibility (fair market value [FMV] assessment and as a % of net patient revenue)					
	4. Possible location identified					
	5. Draft lease obtained					
	6. Legal review of proposed lease					
	7. Execute lease					
	8. Copy and file lease as necessary					
	9. Identify furnishings, fixtures, and equipment (FF&E) available and needed					
	10. Identify telephone system to be used					
	11. Identify electrical, data, and communication ports on floor plans					
	12. Identify electrical needs for outside signage. Obtain and install.					
	13. Arrange for utilities					
	14. Identify and install security system					
	15. Installation of fixed assets					
	16. Arrange for contracted facility services • Answering service • Waste management • Reference lab • Uniform cleaning service • Document shredding service • Housekeeping • Medical records copying service					

Source: The Halley Consulting Group, LLC (www.halleyconsulting.com), copyright

Marketing and Promotion	Action	Project Coordinator	Target Date	Start Date	Completion Date	Notes
Marketing and Promotion	1. Identify signage needs					
	2. Create brochures					
	3. Identify community advertising opportunities for new clinics					
	4. Run newspaper ads for clinic opening					
	5. Assist with web site development					
	6. Identify physician self-promotion activities, i.e., health fairs, speaking opportunities, etc.					

Operational Systems	Action	Project Coordinator	Target Date	Start Date	Completion Date	Notes
Operational Systems	1. Select and order FF&E					
	2. Select and order information systems (IS) equipment					
	3. Establish fee schedules					
	4. Establish Central Business Office Structure and Policies					
	5. Order business supplies					
	6. Create and order charge slips, charting forms, and billing forms					
	7. Order medical business forms and charting materials					
	8. Order reference manuals					
	9. Order medical supplies					

Source: The Halley Consulting Group, LLC (www.halleyconsulting.com), copyright © 2006. Reprinted with permission.

Information Systems	Action	Project Coordinator	Target Date	Start Date	Completion Date	Notes
Information Systems	1. See Appendix I, "Potential Requirements for Mission-Critical Applications."					
	2. Identify potential practice management system vendors. (Determine if electronic health record [EHR] is to be included.)					
	3. Schedule vendor demonstrations.					
	4. Request an RFP from the preferred vendor.					
	5. System selection and contract negotiated for IS system.					
	6. Implementation team to be established.					
	7. Identify implementation action plan and timelines.					

Source: The Halley Consulting Group, LLC (www.halleyconsulting.com), copyright © 2006. Reprinted with permission.

APPENDIX F

Sample Communication Matrix

[Health Care Facility Name]

[Street Address]

[City, ST ZIP Code]

[Phone]

Key Communication Goals and Messages

Goals

1. Support smooth **implementation of the key elements of strategy** as defined by (client) and outlined in the Network Evaluation.
2. **Build** clinic physician and employee engagement for the change process.
3. Create continuous **feedback communication expectations and opportunities** to the Implementation team throughout the entire rollout process.
4. Assure continuous and consistent awareness of the overall objective of "Net 1 Break Even" of (client) clinics by the agreed upon goal of (client).

Messages

1. (Client) clinics face an urgent business imperative to meet financial goals in order to further clinical excellence, safety goals and clinic viability. Measurement and accountability are key to reaching goals.
   a. Dynamic and challenging health care market place
   b. Identified key business needs and challenges as outlined in the Network Evaluation
   c. Identified business imperatives: "net 1" break-even for established clinics
   d. Continued use of audits and reviews of finance, compliance, coding/ documentation practices
   e. No immediate plans to close clinics
   f. Senior leadership endorsement by CEO
   g. (Client) values will guide planning and implementation

---

2. (Client) clinics play a primary role in attracting/retaining customers for the entire (client) delivery system.
   a. Retail strategy repositions and supports (client) clinics to serve as front door for (client) hospitals.
   b. Patient care and access continue to be top priorities.
   c. (Client) will analyze primary retail market share and create strategies to measure, retain and expand market share.
   d. Enhanced focus on training will support clinic providers and staff.
   e. A facilities evaluation and improvement plan will support patient safety, comfort and provider/staff productivity.

3. In order for (client) to meet its strategic goals, (client) must change to work more effectively with clinicians as partners and leaders regarding its strategic and business goals.
   a. New leadership structures (e.g., Network Operations Council) will support physician partnership, influence and accountability through strategy and policy development, and will include physician leadership and involvement.
   b. Physician leaders will continue to be involved in, and will focus further on, clinic governance and support of retail strategy.
   c. Communication of practice goals and measurement will support hospitals in meeting strategic and operational objectives.
   d. All Provider recruitment or practice additions will be evaluated through strategic criteria and transition plans.
   e. Clinic managers and physicians will become very involved in planning for financial performance improvement and will meet regularly.
   f. (Client) clinics will introduce a more complete orientation model, to include mentors for each new provider.
   g. (Client) clinics will place its highest operation priority on supporting the productivity of providers.

Source: The Halley Consulting Group, LLC (www.halleyconsulting.com), copyright © 2005. Reprinted with permission.

Audience	Update	Timing and Frequency	Responsible Party	Medium and Tools
Executive Team	✔ Accountability for Executive Director, etc. ✔ Timing ✔ Action Plans ✔ Communication Matrix framework ✔ Governance Council policy and process	October and periodic updates		Meetings
Implementation Team	✔ Review of Communication Matrix and feedback on audiences, messages and tactics ✔ Assuring the full implementation of the Communication plan elements	October and ongoing on a weekly basis		Complete: met with the team on 11/1 and reviewed Matrix. To review weekly
Clinic Management Team	✔ Governance council role and function ✔ Executive Director accountable for operations ✔ Listening sessions to hear feedback on messages already delivered ✔ Key Goals and Messages 1–3	October		Complete: met with team on 10/17 and reviewed Goals and Messages
Hospital Key Management Team Members	✔ Messages 1–3 ✔ Announcement of position changes: Executive Director, central staff, etc. ✔ Emphasis on transition planning: no clinic closures planned, (client) values	October and periodic updates		Meeting(s)
Clinic Staff	✔ Messages 1–3 ✔ Announcement of position changes: Executive Director, Lead MDs ✔ Emphasis on transition planning: no clinic closures planned, (client) values ✔ Regular updates as needed	3–4 weeks of meetings		Meetings and regular communication updates by site

Source: The Halley Consulting Group, LLC (www.halleyconsulting.com), copyright © 2005. Reprinted with permission.

Audience	Update	Timing and Frequency	Responsible Party	Medium and Tools
Accounting & Finance Mgmt.	✔ Messages 1–3 ✔ Emphasis on Financial reporting requirements and HCG financial model basics and timeline ✔ Management organizational structure	October		Meeting(s)
Medical Staff	✔ Messages 1–3 ✔ Emphasis on 3 (clinicians as partners, leaders)	October		Meetings and/or written communication
Recruitment/ Retention	✔ Messages 1–3 ✔ Emphasis on impact to areas with cross hospital functional responsibility	October		Complete
Clinic Providers By Site (Physicians, Physician Assistants, Nurse Practitioners)	✔ Overview messages 1–3 ✔ Emphasis on 3 ✔ Follow up announcements (as needed)	October and ongoing		Clinic-based meetings, Q & A
Employees	✔ Overview messages 1–3 ✔ New leadership roles ✔ Transition timelines ✔ Emphasize (client) values	October and ongoing		Written weekly publication
Billing Office	✔ Overview messages 1–3 ✔ Review Central Processing Office (CPO) model basics and timeline	October and periodic updates		Meetings
Corporate Board(s)	✔ Overview messages 1–3 ✔ Emphasis on measurement, accountability, provider leadership	October or next available meeting		Board written communication and/or Board Agenda
New Network Operations Council and Local Practice Operations Councils	✔ Status of ongoing work ✔ Action Plan review	Monthly		Meeting attendance

Source: The Halley Consulting Group, LLC (www.halleyconsulting.com), copyright © 2005. Reprinted with permission.

APPENDIX G

Specialist-of-Choice Practice Evaluation

Referral Source Knowledge	● Yes ○ No
1. We have identified all of the potential referring physicians and other providers in our defined geographic market.	○
2. We track volumes by referring physician/provider each month and identify any significant changes.	○
3. We have a written profile for each of our referring physicians and other providers documenting their contact information, any preferences or unique practice characteristics, their office manager or clinical coordinator and other key contacts, and their preferred method and timing for receiving feedback from us.	○
4. We send a brief satisfaction and information gathering survey to the office manager along with the practice holiday gift each year.	○
5. Our physicians, management and staff routinely discuss the results of our surveys and develop action plans to address practice problems and to take advantage of positive suggestions.	○
Referral Source Knowledge: Total Capabilities Identified = (Count Each ● Yes)	

Source: The Halley Consulting Group, LLC (www.halleyconsulting.com), copyright © 2008. Reprinted with permission.

Referral Source Access	● Yes ○ No
6. We have a designated telephone line(s) for referring physicians and other providers to use when contacting our practice or physicians.	○
7. We have assigned an experienced and service-oriented staff member to answer the referring physician line(s) and respond to inquiries from referring physicians and their staff members.	○
8. We accommodate all requests for non-acute appointments within three days.	○
9. We accommodate all referring physician/provider requests for acute appointments each day.	○
10. We have privileges at the hospitals and facilities preferred by our referring physicians/providers.	○
11. Our payer participation matches that of our referring physicians/providers.	○
12. Our office is accessible during all normal business hours, whether the physician/provider is present or not.	○
13. Our call coverage network is comprised of competent associates who share our customer service philosophy toward patients and toward our referring physicians and other providers.	○
14. Our physicians respond to every call from a referring physician's/provider's office within the same day.	○
15. Our physicians provide their pager numbers to key referring physicians/providers for "quick consults."	○
16. We accept all patients and payers from our referring physicians and other providers.	○
17. We provide our fair portion of care for the uninsured and underinsured.	○
18. We provide all pre-authorization services for our patients and referring physicians/providers.	○
19. We have the ability to assist patients in identifying and obtaining alternative funding if they are not insured.	○
20. Our partners and/or mid-level providers handle acute cases that our physicians cannot work into their schedules.	○
21. In regional settings, we provide outreach services to satellites in small communities with primary care physicians/providers and a community hospital.	○
Referral Source Access: Total Capabilities Identified = (Count Each ● Yes)	

Source: The Halley Consulting Group, LLC (www.halleyconsulting.com), copyright © 2008. Reprinted with permission.

Referral Source Expectations	● Yes ○ No
22. When possible and clinically appropriate, our referring physicians and other providers are aware of the routine ancillary tests we need in order to evaluate their patients. They have the option to provide those tests themselves, in which case we always acknowledge and request those test results.	○
23. For patients whose physicians/providers do not provide ancillary services, we will take responsibility to schedule and facilitate the testing prior to the first visit, if necessary.	○
24. We make an information package available to referring offices to share with patients. The package includes maps, welcome information, and instructions for patients who are referred to us.	○
25. We provide the ancillary services routinely expected of our specialty according to the community standard of care.	○
Referral Source Expectations: Total Capabilities Identified = (Count Each ● Yes)	

Customer Service Team	● Yes ○ No
26. We hire outgoing, friendly staff members who view "customer" service as part of their personal mission in life, whether that customer is a patient, a family member, a referring physician/provider or staff member.	○
27. Our current staff members recommend new hires they think will "fit" our customer-focused culture.	○
28. Staff members are trained to respond to physicians/providers and their staff members as very critical customers.	○
29. Each of our staff members receives formal training in customer service techniques.	○
30. All staff members go through a formal customer service training process annually.	○
31. Customer service is one of the critical factors in every staff member's performance appraisal.	○
32. All of our staff members are well trained in their technical role within the practice. Trainees are identified for our retail customers and do not manage the referring physician telephone line.	○
Customer Service Team: Total Capabilities Identified = (Count Each ● Yes)	

Relationship Management	●Yes ○No
33. According to the referring physician's/provider's profile and preference, we teleconference and/or provide written feedback on each new referral within 24 hours of initial evaluation.	○
34. We acknowledge the referring physician or other provider to the patient during each patient encounter.	○
35. Whenever possible, and according to the referring physician/provider profile, we refer our patients back to their primary care physician/provider for follow up care. This verbal "referral" is accompanied by a referral form copied to the referring physician's/provider's office.	○
36. We acknowledge the role of non-physician primary care providers and value them as customers.	○
37. We offer to conference with the referring physician/provider while the patient is in the examination room, according to the physician's/provider's profile.	○
38. We communicate with the referring physician or other provider within 24 hours after any significant event, surgery or procedure. According to the physician's/provider's profile, this communication may be a telephone call, email or letter.	○
39. We routinely communicate with the referring physician or other provider during the course of treatment of a chronically ill patient according to the profile.	○
40. We ensure that there is adequate coordination of care for each patient referred to us either through their primary care physician/provider, hospitalist, or our office. This coordination includes, at a minimum, pain management and medication management.	○
41. We include complimentary specialty physicians in our relationship development and management activities, to ensure that we function as a team to meet the needs, wants, and priorities of our referring physicians/providers and their patients.	○
42. Our profile contains each referring physician's/provider's preferred hospital and we contact that physician or provider before performing a procedure in any other facility.	○
43. We chart and initial every interaction with a referring physician's/provider's office.	○
44. We survey each referred patient and obtain their permission to share the results with their referring physician.	○
45. We participate in leadership positions to strengthen the local medical staff of hospitals where we have active staff privileges. As part of our leadership role, we acknowledge and protect the interests of our referring physicians/providers.	○
46. During telephone contact with a referring physician/provider or their staff, we routinely ask "how" our service to them and their patients could be enhanced.	○
47. Any negative feedback received from a referring physician/provider or referred patient is addressed in regular meetings with a written response going to both the referring physician/provider and the patient, as appropriate.	○
Relationship Management: Total Capabilities Identified = (Count Each ● Yes)	

Source: The Halley Consulting Group, LLC (www.halleyconsulting.com), copyright © 2008. Reprinted with permission.

Education/Promotion	●Yes ○No
48. We support our referring physicians/providers by making available high quality educational information for their patients regarding common ailments or conditions specific to our practice specialty.	○
49. We volunteer to provide lectures and education to assist primary care physicians/providers in becoming more knowledgeable and effective in their clinical practice in our area of expertise.	○
50. We acknowledge our referring physicians/providers and their office staff with an additional token of our appreciation during the Holiday season.	○
Education/Promotion: Total Capabilities Identified = (Count Each ● Yes)	

Specialist of Choice **Practice Evaluation Scores** (Transfer totals from previous sections)	
Referral Source Knowledge	
Referral Source Access	
Referral Source Expectations	
Customer Service Team	
Relationship Management	
Education/Promotion	
Total	
Overall Score + 50 × 100 = (Rounded to the nearest whole number)	

Source: The Halley Consulting Group, LLC (www.halleyconsulting.com), copyright

APPENDIX H

Medical Practice Clinical Productivity Evaluation

Clinical Setting	Yes	No
1. Does each physician have at least three dedicated patient examination rooms?		
2. Are examination rooms arranged and stocked similarly?		
3. Is there standardization of medical record construct and forms among physicians?		
4. Is pertinent and current medical information always contained within the medical record for each patient visit?		
5. Are office meetings, in-service meetings, and drug representatives scheduled during non-patient times?		
6. Is the patient schedule managed properly so that "no-shows" are less than 5 percent of all appointments?		
7. Are time slots allocated in the morning and afternoon for same day/work-in appointments?		
8. Does each physician have a permanently assigned clinical assistant?		
9. Is the clinical assistant always in or within sight of the examination rooms?		
10. Is the clinical assistant charged with the responsibility to manage the physician's productivity, including monitoring exam room time and moving the physician along, as appropriate?		
11. Is the clinical assistant responsible for patient education and patient discharge instructions?		
12. Is physician productivity recognized as a major job function for all staff members?		
13. Is physician productivity a standing item on staff meeting agendas?		
14. Do patients complain about excessive reception area or examination room wait times?		
15. Are pulmonary function studies, spirometry, breathing treatments, routine blood pressure checks, venipunctures, EKGs, family consultations, extended patient counseling, or other similar services performed in a patient examination room?		
16. Does the provider experience downtime waiting for patients to be assigned/triaged to the examination room?		
17. Does the practice experience overtime on a routine basis because patient visits run late?		
18. Does the clinical assistant spend time on the phone while the physician is seeing scheduled patients?		

Scoring: Total the number of responses from this section and indicate the number below

A. Questions 1–13. Indicate the number of "Yes" answers ______________

B. Questions 14–18. Indicate the number of "No" answers ______________

Total Clinical Setting Score (A + B) ______________

Source: The Halley Consulting Group, LLC (www.halleyconsulting.com), copyright © 2008. Reprinted with permission.

Physician Personal Productivity	Yes	No
19. Does the physician start each appointment block on time?		
20. Does the physician double book patients on a daily basis?		
21. Does the physician dictate/record progress notes at the close of each visit?		
22. Has the physician approved policies and procedures to define the process for prescription refills, patient care inquiries, laboratory panic values, etc.?		
23. Are patient scheduling templates created to support individual physician productivity as opposed to a "one template fits all" mentality? (For example, can the software accommodate a block schedule, wave schedule and modified wave schedule?)		
24. Does the current technology support physician productivity (e.g., electronic medical record, PDA, email, Internet access, etc.)?		
25. Does the physician's personal productivity account for at least 30 percent of his or her personal income?		
26. Does the physician routinely fall more than 15 minutes behind schedule?		
27. Does the physician schedule more than 30 minutes for any office visit?		
28. Does the physician address every complaint of the patient during the visit (as opposed to just those for which the patient is scheduled)?		
29. Does the physician allow interruptions while in the examination room to respond to patient, physician, or hospital telephone calls?		
30. Does the physician periodically cancel patients for non-emergent reasons?		

Scoring: Total the number of responses from this section and indicate the number below

C. Questions 19–25. Indicate the number of "Yes" answers __________

D. Questions 26–30. Indicate the number of "No" answers __________

Total Physician Personal Productivity Score (C + D) __________

Circle the total score for each section in the graphs below

Clinical Setting Score

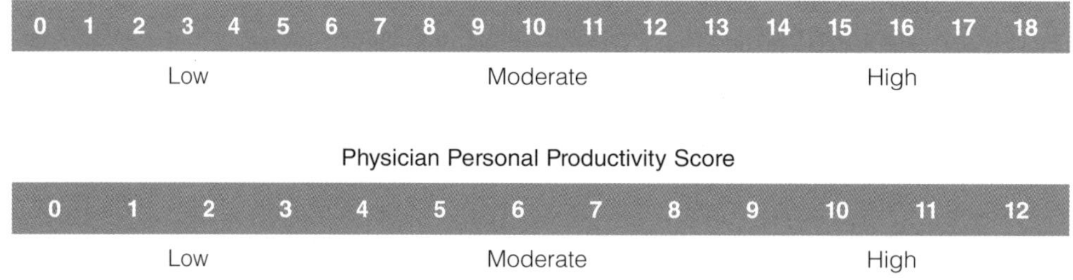

Source: The Halley Consulting Group, LLC (www.halleyconsulting.com), copyright © 2008. Reprinted with permission.

APPENDIX I

Potential Requirements for Mission-Critical Applications

Item	PM*	EHR*	Required	Desired	Optional
FUNCTIONALITY—CLINICAL					
Alerts (e.g., drug interactions, chronic diagnoses)					
Clinical best practice indicators and decision support					
Supports back-office work flow (e.g., patients checked in and waiting)					
Charting					
Charting customization (e.g., by provider, by specialty)					
Orders/computerized physician order entry (CPOE)					
Triage nurse support					
Electronic prescriptions					
Diagnostic test results					
Digital image review					
Chronic diagnosis management					
Clinical progress/outcomes reporting					
Reports and clinical data mining					
Support for the Physician Quality Reporting Initiative (PQRI)					
Others . . .					

*PM = practice management system; EHR = electronic health record (often called electronic medical record).

Source: The Halley Consulting Group, LLC (www.halleyconsulting.com), copyright © 2008. Reprinted with permission.

Item	PM*	EHR*	Required	Desired	Optional
FUNCTIONALITY—CLERICAL					
Patient database mining by demographics, by diagnosis, etc.					
Telephone switchboard support (e.g., appointment scheduling, triage nurse)					
Appointment scheduling (e.g., patient access, centralized, decentralized)					
Insurance pre-authorization					
Registration					
Patient cycle time (e.g., wait time by location)					
Managing paper, scans, faxes					
Office suite (e.g., e-mail, word processing, spreadsheets, presentations)					
Reports and queries (e.g., standard and custom)					
Others . . .					
FUNCTIONALITY—REVENUE CYCLE					
Patients self–check in					
Data verification: required fields					
Insurance verification					
Co-payment request and processing					
Patient cycle time (e.g., wait time alerts)					
Fee ticket or "super bill" generation					
Procedure and diagnosis coding support					
Cashier function (e.g., patient-due balances)					
Central processing office functions					
Others . . .					
SYSTEM					
Administration: how features, privileges, and permissions of the system are set up and maintained					
Audit trail: data entry and data changes, electronic signature					
Bandwidth: volume, capacity, peaks, redundancy, contingency for outage (more bandwidth is needed for hosted approach and remote clinics)					

Source: The Halley Consulting Group, LLC (www.halleyconsulting.com), copyright © 2008. Reprinted with permission.

Item	PM*	EHR*	Required	Desired	Optional
Certification by the Certification Commission for Healthcare Information Technology (CCHIT)					
Data conversion (from existing system): the process; the support needed from the existing system and vendor; typical time frame to convert from an existing system					
Hardware requirements: for each user (laptop, tablet, hand-held); servers (if not vendor hosted); peripherals for each work group or location (printers, fax, medical equipment)					
Compliance with the Health Insurance Portability and Accountability Act of 1996 (HIPAA)					
Infrastructure: located at the practice level or centralized for the entire network; hosted by the vendor over the Internet					
Reliability: evaluate reliability, security, backup/recovery, firewall, redundancy					
Installation process: a typical approach; time frame; issues specific to your organization requiring customization					
Maintenance and upgrades: frequency of updates, how they are applied, how they affect your customizations					
Meaningful use: the percentage of current standards met by the software					
Operating system (if not vendor hosted): licenses, upgrades, patches, staff support required to maintain the system locally					
Security: penetration prevention, virus, spam, spyware, malware, firewall					
Security/privileges: established and set by role and individual					
Support available: within the application, online, help desk (how many staff, ratio of staff to customers, scheduled hours, on-call availability), options and costs					
System features: the "look and feel," drop-down menus, quick-fill fields, acceptable values (to reduce errors), number of clicks and screens to accomplish a task, ability to interrupt and resume, intuitive navigation, searching, etc.					
Training: categories of users, duration, approach					
Others . . .					

Source: The Halley Consulting Group, LLC (www.halleyconsulting.com), copyright © 2008. Reprinted with permission.

Item	PM*	EHR*	Required	Desired	Optional
VENDOR GUARANTEES					
Meaningful use qualification					
Supports pay for performance (P4P)					
Provider productivity levels: the time frame to return to previous level and/or increase productivity					
Qualification for federal stimulus bonus payments per provider, based on the Health Information Technology for Economic and Clinical Health Act of 2009 (HITECH)					
Service levels: for installation, training, support					
Uptime: of system in established locations					
Others . . .					
VENDOR QUALIFICATION					
Problem resolution: approach and process to work through the challenges that will arise					
Data ownership: how to retain/access your data in the event of breach of contract					
Financial stability of the vendor					
Reference checks: access to installed customer base					
Site visits: customers similar to your organization					
Terms and conditions: of formal contractual relationship					
Others . . .					
CONSTRAINTS					
Cost: initial purchase and through year 5					
Host: hosted internally (requires servers and staff to maintain) or hosted by vendor					
Interface: must integrate with existing software/systems/equipment (e.g., hospital EHR)					
P4P: level of reporting required					
Performance improvement: identify specific processes to be improved prior to installation, including benchmark and timeline					

Source: The Halley Consulting Group, LLC (www.halleyconsulting.com), copyright © 2008. Reprinted with permission.

Item	PM*	EHR*	Required	Desired	Optional
Return on investment (ROI): required percentage and measures established					
Solution set: single integrated solution (practice management and EHR) versus multiple products from multiple vendors requiring an interface					
Conversion timeline: to convert, train, implement, and transition from existing systems					
Equipment: use of existing equipment (requires a complete equipment inventory); willingness to upgrade existing hardware or to purchase additional capacity; or partial/full replacement					
Others . . .					

COSTS	Year 1	Year 2	Year 3	Year 4	Year 5
Configuration: acceptable values, field names, screen labels, specialty uniqueness					
Customization: fields, screens, work flow					
Data conversion/migration: from existing systems					
Infrastructure: hardware, software, operating systems, broadband					
Licenses: by site, provider, user (named or concurrent), volume, month/quarter					
Maintenance and upgrades					
Payment: options					
Support: types and levels					
Training: initial (on-site, groups of users, super user, administrator), performance improvement, troubleshooting					
Others . . .					

Source: The Halley Consulting Group, LLC (www.halleyconsulting.com), copyright © 2008. Reprinted with permission.

Index

D

E

F

G

H